MEDICAL
BIOMAGNETISM

Illustrated: 351 Treatment Pairs

A Visual Guide of Dr. Isaac Goiz Duran's
Revolutionary Medical Legacy

VICTORIA VIVALDI

MEDICAL
BIOMAGNETISM

Illustrated: 351 Treatment Pairs

A Visual Guide of Dr. Isaac Goiz Duran's
Revolutionary Medical Legacy

VICTORIA VIVALDI

For questions or comments regarding this book, please contact:
Email: *VictoriaVivaldiBooks@gmail.com*

ISBN: 9781791617080 (paperback)
Independently published

Design elements:
Designed by Freepile and vecteezy.com

Children see water as water, trees as trees,
and mountains as mountains...
Students see water as chemistry, trees as dendrology,
and mountains as orography...
The *studied, old and wise* see water as water, trees as trees,
and mountains as mountains...

(-Adapted by V. Vivaldi from Quingyuan Weixing, 9th century)

DISCLAIMER

The information provided in this book is for general informational purposes only. The author and publisher make no representations or warranties of any kind, express or implied, about the suitability, reliability, or applicability of the information contained within these pages.

The techniques, practices, and suggestions presented in this book are not intended as a substitute for professional advice, diagnosis, or treatment. Readers should consult with qualified professionals in the respective fields regarding any specific concerns or issues they may have. The author and publisher disclaim any liability for damages or losses directly or indirectly arising from the use or application of any information provided in this book.

Furthermore, the mention or inclusion of any third-party resources, websites, or products in this book does not constitute an endorsement or recommendation. Readers are responsible for conducting their own research and due diligence before making any decisions or utilizing any external resources mentioned.

The views expressed by the author in this book are solely their own and do not necessarily reflect the views of the publisher or any other individuals or organizations associated with the book.

The content of this book is subject to change and may be updated or revised periodically. The author and publisher reserve the right to modify or discontinue any aspect of this book at any time without prior notice.

Reading and implementing the information provided in this book is at the reader's own risk. The author and publisher shall not be held liable for any direct, indirect, incidental, consequential, or punitive damages or losses arising from the use or misuse of the information contained in this book.

By reading this book, you acknowledge and agree to the terms and conditions stated in this disclaimer.

TABLE OF CONTENTS

Introduction by Victoria Vivaldi

Growing up, from childhood into adulthood in my mid-30s, my understanding of health and wellness meant that whenever there was any sign of sickness, we must run to the medical doctor for a checkup and get medicine, either as a prescription or over the counter.

This was my belief until one day, after feeling exhausted from feeling chronically miserable for years, having had three surgeries by that point, and taking medication after medication, I decided to seek wellness solutions elsewhere. Being fed up, and taking a different action was the best thing I could have ever done for myself!

After many years of haling medical doctors as is if the acronym M.D. meant *medium deus* (demi god), that was now a long overdue expired belief! And it all started by finally being curious enough to read the insert of my prescription drugs. Surprising enough, the possible side-effects described many of the symptoms I was experiencing at the time.

Looking back, it's so pathetic how when I would bring this up to the attending medical doctor, she was dismissive, simply telling me that there is no correlation between the medicine she was prescribing to my new health issues. I knew then that enough was enough, and that I had to look for alternatives!

I immediately abandoned all medication, and my search took me towards nutrition, herbs and natural supplements. And guess what happened? Within two week, my health had dramatically improved. The acidity, the annoyance, the fatigue and all other symptoms plaguing me completely disappeared.

I strongly believe that had I kept on following the medical doctor's advice, and ignoring my gut feeling (no pun intended), I probably would have ended up with a fourth surgery soon. This was 20 years ago, and I know had I continued this path, I would likely be in a worse situation, especially now considering all the bad medical advice given to us during the *scamdemic*!

Now I'm not telling you any of this to demean doctors. I have nothing against doctors; in fact, I still have periodic medical check-ups for myself and my children.

My story and the essense of this book lie in the recognition that our knowledge is limited. No one possesses all the answers, including myself. What I present to you today is a summary and visual representation of the extraordinary medical legacy left by the late Dr. Isaac Goiz Duran, M.D. He discovered the groundbreaking technique of advanced magnet placement on the body, unlocking effective and powerful healing potentials.

Additionally, I am excited to introduce two new pendulum chart books that perfectly complement this illustrated book and the biomagnetic recalibration methodology developed by Moses Durazo. These pendulum books offer invaluable support to Dr. Goiz's diagnosis and the 6-day recalibration process, enhancing the potential for profound healing and transformation.

I am also bringing focus to the work of Mr. Moses Durazo, a direct disciple of Dr. Goiz Duran. Today, he stands as a trailblazer, propelling the awareness and understanding of Medical and Recalibration Biomagnetism—an avenue that offers safe and natural solutions for holistic well-being. Witnessing Mr. Durazo's dedication and passion for helping others has been a source of immense joy. Both my children and I have personally experienced the effectiveness of this science, utilizing his self-care biomagnetic kits and delving into the wisdom he imparts through his books.

As I delved into Mr. Durazo's references to the late Dr. Goiz, I felt a sense of curiosity and happiness. It is for this reason that I asked to interview Mr. Durazo about what got him into the field, and if he could talk to me more about who Dr. Goiz was as a man and a teacher, and see what other valuable pieces of information we can learn from him.

Fortunately, Mr. Durazo agreed to share his knowledge and experiences. I hope you enjoy this journey as we explore the remarkable contributions of Dr. Goiz Duran. embrace the power of recalibration biomagnetism, and utilize the support of the two new pendulum chart books. Together, they offer a comprehensive approach to healing and well-being that can change your life in extraordinary ways.

2

Durazo's Experience and Advice

Q: *Will you tell us where and when you trained in Medical Pair Biomagnetism?*

A: In 2008, I had the great privilege of traveling to Mexico City to study the *Medical Biomagnetic Pair* science directly with Dr. Isaac Goiz Durán, M.D., who discovered and developed this medical treatment since 1988.

Q: *Why did you choose to study this field?*

A: I decided to train in this field and dedicate myself to helping others with their wellness goals by applying this science, and writing several books about this topic, because this specific biomagnetic therapy changed me forever! And I thought to myself, *if I don't do it, who will?*

Q: *How did it change you?*

A: With *only one* medical biomagnetic pair session, a chronic digestive issue that had been plaguing me for 4 ½ years disappeared overnight. I had tried everything; it wasn't for lack of trying. Mind you, I had completed a holistic health program at the university. But despite all the natural medicine modalities I was trained in, and was applying, and then seeking help from other healthcare professionals, my suffering was *still* unrelenting - the truth was that my extensive training, and that of other practitioners simply was not enough! And now it was finally over!

This biomagnetic experience also changed me by lighting a passion deep within to want to help as many people as I can obtain and maintain optimal wellness. Today, some 15 years later, I have now helped thousands of people transform miserable pain and suffering to wellbeing, simply by using magnets.

Q: *I can definitely relate! Will you explain how this specific type of Biomagnetism works?*

A: Medical Biomagnetic Pair therapy is a means of restoring wellness without the use of medication or surgery. It is a science-based theory that allows us to diagnose and successfully treat many illnesses using pairs of medium-intensity magnets.

The magnets are used specifically to normalize a diseased/imbalanced organism's potential hydrogen (pH) levels. Changes in the pH level of an organ or body system are linked to the presence of viruses, toxins, parasites, fungi and other harmful intruders and stressors in the body.

Q: *What has been people's response to what you do, for example, your family, friends or new people you meet?*

A: Magnets?! People often react in surprise when they learn of my specialty. I definitely understand; I too reacted with surprise and skepticism when I first heard about the benefits of Medical Pair Biomagnetism.

I had first equated "Biomagnetism" with shoe inserts and magnetic jewelry; believe me, in my quest to finding healing, I had already purchased magnetic shoe inserts that I was told yielded great health benefits, but after years of using them, I did not notice any benefit whatsoever...

When it was explained that Biomagnetism can be used to treat and cure serious health issues, now, that just sounded *completely absurd* to me, and I rejected that notion altogether.

Others probably feel the same, but out of politeness, they don't tell it to me directly. I usually hear about the skepticism from people who are so excited about their results, but can't manage to convince friends or family members, who then make fun of them and criticize them for seeking my services.

Q: *What was the process from going from skepticism to now dedicating your life to this biomagnetic mission?*

A: I went from being a closed-minded skeptic to an open-minded skeptic when I was told that the benefits and application of the Biomagnetic Pair science is incomparable to magnetic jewelry or shoe inserts - that I should not even equate them. Something inside of me then nagged me to look more into this topic - I'm pretty sure it was God talking to me. My initial resistance then began to fade, and I started becoming more excited about trying something new, after all, what did I have to lose?

Q: *And did you lose anything as a result of trying Biomagnetism?*

A: Well, depends on how you look at it...I suppose I lost doubt, fear and resistance, and fortunately by acting as an open-minded skeptic, I gained knowledge and experience that only happens by taking action. Today, together with hundreds of thousands of people worldwide who have experienced this natural therapy firsthand, we have become strong voices unified in its praise.

Q: *What do you think would happen if more people tried Biomagnetism?*

A: I strongly believe that the reality would be shocking. If everybody on earth tried this method, pain and suffering would dramatically decrease, the quality of life would be greatly enhanced, and we would save billions, if not trillions of dollars in healthcare costs that support many over-priced treatments that are less effective.

Q: *I believe that just like me, more and more people are waking up to the failed tragedy of modern day allopathic medicine as governed by corrupt bodies, and people want to reclaim their individual power. What is your thought about this?*

A: I agree with you. More and more people want to *steer clear* of medical visits, and avoid getting sucked into the ever spinning hamster wheel of pills, testing, more pills, more testing, surgery, more pills, lotions, potions and an abundance of fear, frustration and powerlessness to dictate ones path.

Don't get me wrong, there is a time and place for all of the above, but the truth is, more and more people are discovering and wanting to live in their God-given power! I believe that together, we may achieve a greater quality of life, simply by incorporating magnets into our way of life!

Q: *What is your opinion about the public health agencies's pandemic response?*

A: My teacher and mentor, Dr. Isaac Goiz, M.D. told us 15 years ago in training that what we are experiencing today (back then) is an obsolete and inefficient medical system that is desperately trying to hold on to power - basing his conclusion on the level of persecution against him from the authorities. Today's draconian public health measures that are clearly not rooted in legitimate science only highlight Dr. Goiz' comments...and I'd love to talk more about this if you'd like.

Q: *I would definitely like to know more about Dr. Goiz. My intention is to document this conversation in a book, and to share Dr. Goiz' teachings to the world by illustrating Medical Pair Biomagnetism. What are your thoughts about this project? Any suggestions?*

A: I commend you for doing your part in helping the world through your actions. I'm sure it will be impactful. Having written six books, I would suggest that your book serve as an easy to understand reference, as opposed to attempting to summarize the totality of Dr. Goiz' teachings .

Q: *If Dr. Goiz were alive, do you think he would approve?*

A: I started writing books precisely because he asked us to document and write about our biomagnetic experiences. I think he would approve if the information provided was accurate and well-intended.

I remember in training Dr. Goiz singling out a specific book and author. He wasn't shy about expressing his disdain for this individual. I'm not interested in singling out this book here today with you, so please don't ask about it...All I will say is that it's a popular book, with great online reviews, but the truth is that the author got most of his teachings wrong. You know, you have to be really careful about fake news nowadays!

For many years, I thought Dr. Goiz had exaggerated his contempt towards this author. But as I decided to write my own books, I looked to that book as part of my research. I finally understood Dr. Goiz' frustration. As someone who keeps as true to his teachings as possible, that book is a hot mess!

Q: *Can you help me understand where the author of this book went wrong so I may avoid the same mistake?*

A: I think the author of that book metaphorically bit off more than she could chew. I'm only assuming here, but maybe she didn't understand Spanish well enough to comprehend Dr. Goiz' lectures and/or books.

She attempted to write a teach-all book, and it simply is not to professional biomagnetic standards.

Through personal experience, I and my professional colleagues can tell you that to master Medical Pair Biomagnetism, you absolutely require proper hands-on instruction from a professional, so please don't mislead people into believing they are going to master Medical Pair Biomagnetism because they have a book in their hands!

Q: *Your points are well taken! Can we now talk more about your direct experience with Dr. Goiz?*

A: Sure, ask all you want...!

REMEMBERING DR. GOIZ

Q: *In as short a summary as possible, what is your memory of Dr. Goiz?*

A: Dr. Isaac Goiz Durán, M.D. was a great and captivating speaker. He was kind, yet temperamental and condescending. If he were a dish, I would say, *sweet and sour*.

He would talk of many things beyond the topics of medicine, but tie those topics into our human experiences. His narratives were captivating, heart-moving, inspirational and even shocking, intimidating and infuriating.

Q: *What are some of the most impacting stories you remember?*

A: In general summary, he would speak of:

• How allopathic medicine had horrifically failed his mother, who passed away in his adolescence. The effects of the torturous bouts of chemotherapy, radiation, surgical intervention and heavy drugging all combined, appeared to him worse than the disease itself. I still remember his eyes swell, and his voice shake in sadness as he recounted this experience.

• How his father, who was also a medical doctor, felt impotent to save his wife, and after her death, abandoned his medical practice. Dr. Goiz stated that his father ended up devoting himself to a spiritual life.

• How the emotional pain of losing his mother and seeing his father's rejection of allopathic medicine was the impetus to embarking on a medical journey intent on improving medicine by also being open to natural medicine possibilities...which by the way, sounds like our own experiences, right...?

• How in 1988 he received a *divine* message about the use of magnets for healing.

• How Dr. Richard Broeringmeyer's biomagnetic field research influenced him, and how he began to wonder, *"If you can detect pH distortions using medium intensity field magnets, then can you correct them as well?!"*

• How incredibly frustrating it was to be ignored by the medical and public health authorities about his *biomagnetic pair* discovery, even though his clinical evidence of efficacy healing documented ill patients mounted.

• How stressful it was to be persecuted by the medical system for going against the "official" medical narrative of the departments of public health. In fact, he would often interject, *"Heal and be quiet!"*, so as to not bring unwanted attention from the tyrants in authority.

• How demoralizing it was to discover that the World Health Organization (WHO) is also complicit in maintaining a for profit bio-pharmaceutical-complex healthcare system that is undermining access to safe, natural and effective medicine to humanity as a whole, and he would talk about so much more...

Q: *Okay, wow, all of these are big topics! Going back to Dr. Goiz' statement of, "The cure being worse than the disease" strikes a nerve for me as it relates to the blundered global pandemic response that has and continues to hurt us financially, and harm us health wise, as the vaccine injury side-effects data is indicating. Do you have anything to say about this?*

A: In today's COVID era, it is blatantly obvious that the allopathic medical system, their governing bodies, along with the media, have grossly failed the scientific method and decent human morality, but the truth is that this has been going on for many years. It just so happens that it is now blatantly in our face!

Q: *What do you think Dr. Goiz would say about what's going on today?*

A: I think he would say that there is nothing new under the heavens and the sun. The fact is that he, and all other great minds throughout history, face resistance from the current powers that be; it just so happens he started dealing with it since 1988 when he discovered the biomagnetic pair application and he wanted the world to benefit from his discovery.

Dr. Goiz told us about an instance where the World Health Organization (WHO) was offering a large money-prize to whomever developed either a cure or treatment for HIV/AIDS. He submitted his thesis titled, **AIDS is Curable** (El SIDA es Curable).

He recalled getting a call from the WHO inviting him to Geneva, and went on to say:

> *"And here goes stupid Goiz, thinking I won the prize, only to be told, 'if what you are claiming here is true, then who is going to pay for all of this* [laboratory]*?'*

What Dr. Goiz was saying is that his biomagnetic treatment discovery produced zero dividends and could not maintain their laboratory expenses. He went on to relate that they handed him his thesis and application check and sent him away...I suppose such an anti-scientific and morally deficient rejection can only be said in person...

Q: *Incredible! What more did he say about this?*

A: Dr. Goiz was driving the point that the authorities know that wellness solutions exist, and that they are running a business that has no room for natural medicine - period!

Q: *And what happened after this?*

A: Dr. Goiz stated that he made it his mission to teach Biomagnetism to whoever would listen. He said he originally intended to teach medical doctors exclusively, but they were not interested. They thought of him as a medical quack. And that those medical doctors that were curious enough to listen, didn't bother practicing Biomagnetism because there is no money to be made by curing people. It's ongoing prescriptions, tests after tests, and surgeries that keep the steady flow of income flowing in that system...

Q: *So if nobody would really listen to him, how did he become so famous?*

A: Because he began teaching people like you and me, who are open to natural holistic medicine, and word spread, and he would then teach laypeople, and even began going to remote villages throughout Latin-America to teach indigenous communities to be self-sufficient.

Q: *Is it true that today, the country of Ecuador is probably the only country where medical doctors and biomagnetic specialists work side-by-side in hospital and clinical settings.*

A: My understanding is the government and the people of that country have their medical system rooted both in allopathy and natural cultural medicines, and Medical Pair Biomagnetism was quickly embraced!

Q: *Is there any proof that Biomagnetism works, and how do people find it?*

A: Proof that it works is everywhere. Simply in the fact that universities have adopted Dr. Goiz teachings, and the increasing number of practitioners worldwide, and people curing and improving using this science should be evidence enough.

In or around 2009, Dr. Raymond Hilu and Dr. Isaac Goiz Durán conducted a before and after study using darkfield microscopy with hundreds of patients who were previously documented as having illness and/or disease.

The changes in the quality of blood of each patient was immediately identified, for which Dr. Hilu stated that without a doubt, Dr. Goiz should be awarded a Nobel Peace Prize, and hopefully, one day soon it will be posthumously awarded.

Q: *Because people are so skeptical, is there anything you can say to convince anybody to try Biomagnetism?*

A: I learned many years ago that people build greater resistance and resentment when you try to convince them of something. Just notice how emotionally charged religious, and political conversations can get - the topic of allopathic versus natural medicine is no different.

I agreed to this conversation with you because the best I can do is deliver my truthful experience, and hopefully my experience helps someone explore Biomagnetism even further. And so long as I have life, my mission is to help those that seek and are ready to receive help.

Q: *Your directness is much appreciated! What else would you like to talk about?*

A: Well, because you are going to provide people with an illustrated guide, it is very likely that people will get their biomagnetic kits - and hopefully they use the ones from SaveMeMagnets.com - I hope you don't mind the plug. Also, I think it's important that you make clear how to read the illustrations, and to make sure people understand the contraindications.

ILLUSTRATIONS AND CONTRAINDICATIONS

I n the following pages, the illustrations are marked with diamond shapes on the anatomical locations where both a positive and a negative magnetic field are placed.

You will notice that these diamond shapes do not indicate which anatomical structure requires the positive or negative field. That is simply because the distorted pH of those tissues may require one polarity or the other. That is determined by biomagnetic or bioenergetic diagnosing; you may visit www.SaveMeMagnets.com for biomagnetic/bioenergetic diagnosing courses.

In the following pages, biomagnetic pairings are organized based on their type, such as for: *virus, bacteria, fungi, parasites, dysfunctions, reservoirs,* and the *special* type.

Regarding special pairs, Dr. Goiz had labeled them by people's names. In this guide, for the sake of getting straight to the point, they are simply described for their corrective function or what they identify (indicate), for example, a special pair that helps correct or improve *ectopic pregnancy* or *tinnitus*, or a special pair that *indicates pregnancy*.

CONTRAINDICATION 1: *out of all existing pairs, the pregnancy indication pair* (Uterus/Ovary) *is the only one that will **NEVER** be applied.* This pair simply identifies that due to pregnancy, the pH of these two environments has changed, which is verifiable through the diagnostic process.

Reason: <u>Application of this biomagnetic pair may neutralize the pH of these anatomical structures and thereby potentially terminate the pregnancy</u>.

Understand, however, that Biomagnetism may be used during pregnancy. Pregnant women all over the world have and continue to incorporate Biomagnetism as part of their prenatal care.

CONTRAINDICATION 2: *Do NOT apply Medical Biomagnetism to people CURRENTLY undergoing chemotherapy.*

Reason 1: Biomagnetism helps with overall body function, thus the chemotherapy absorbtion to the cells may greatly increase, thereby potentially amplifying intoxication- and other adverse side-effects.

Suggestion: Wait at least one month after the last chemotherapy treatment prior to engaging in the application of Biomagnetic Pair treatments.

Reason 2: For your own peace of mind. Dr. Goiz would remind us that people and family members often want to blame someone when a person feels worse and/or passes away, so it's better to not get involved.

CONTRAINDICATION 3*: Do NOT put magnets directly over an electronic implant, such as pacemakers, medicine releasing devices or other.*

Reason 1: Batteries drain faster when exposed to magnetism.

Reason 2: Magnetism may alter the device's settings.

Understand, however, that Biomagnetism may be used when people do have these electronic and especially non-electronic implants, such as metal plates, screws and other.

GENERAL PHARMACEUTICAL SUGGESTION: be actively aware of how you are feeling and/or your body-function/sign measurements, such as blood sugar or pressure levels. If you notice radical and/or concerning shifts, immediately consult with your medical doctor to see if the pharmaceutical dosages must be reduced (which is tipically the case).

Reason: better body function means less medication. The same holds true for natural supplementation - you may need less supplements.

Viral Infection Pairs

Adenovirus
Hepatic Ligament - Kidney (Right)

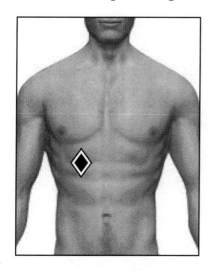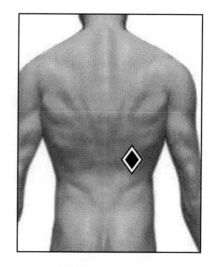

Adenovirus
Pancreas - Pancreas

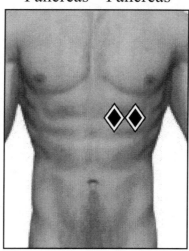

ADENOVIRUS 33
Adrenal - Oblongata

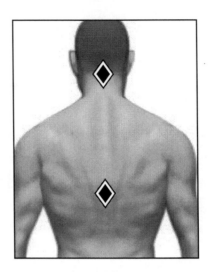

AFTOSA/FOOT AND MOUTH
Thoracic 3 - Thoracic 7

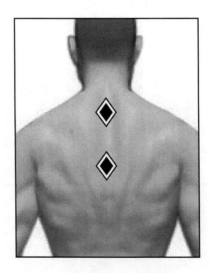

AH1N7
Gallbladder - Spleen

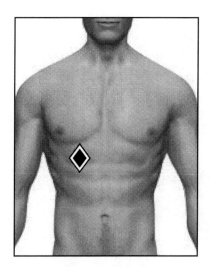 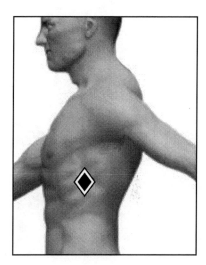

ANISAKIASIS VIRUS
Pancreas Tail - Decending Colon

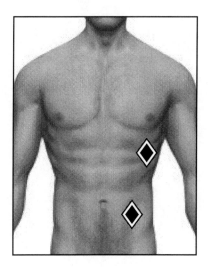

APHTOSE FEVER
Carina - Carina

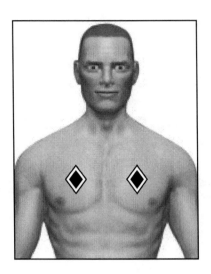

BKV
Appendix - Kidney (Left)

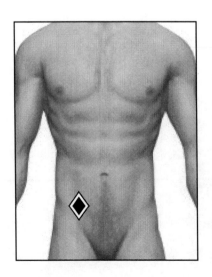
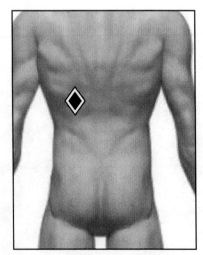

CHIKUNGUNYA
Descending Colon - Anus

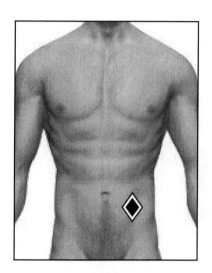 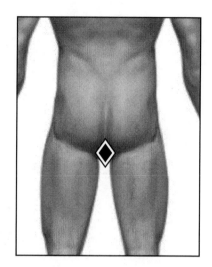

COMMON COLD
Gallbladder - Kidney (Right)

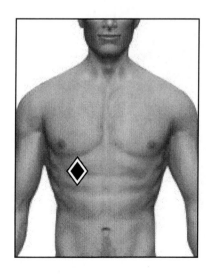 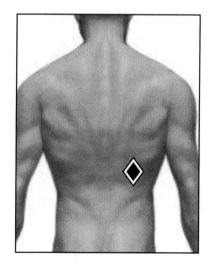

COMMON SKIN TAG
Pancreas Tip - Spleen

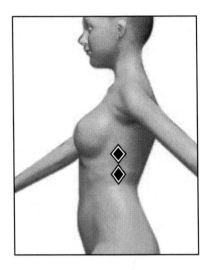

CORONAVIRUS
Urethra - Urethra

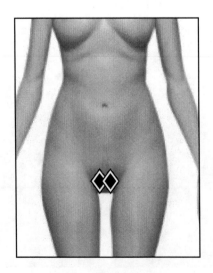

COXSACKIEVIRUS
Sternum Handle - Sternum Handle

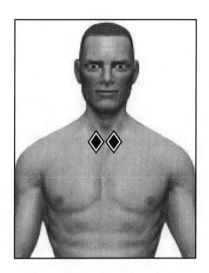

CYTOMEGALOVIRUS
Eye - Eye

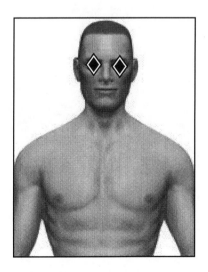

DENGUE
Pituitary - Bladder

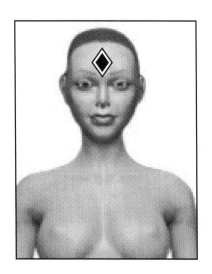 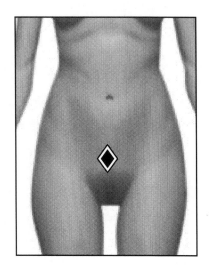

EBOLA
Costal (anterior) - Costal (anterior)

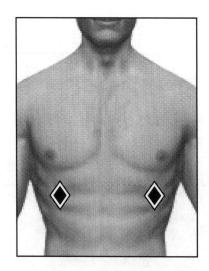

ENTEROVIRUS
Malar - Malar

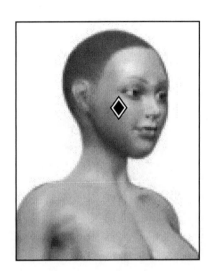
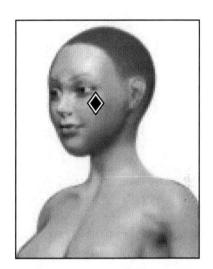

EPSTEIN-BARR
Occipital - Occipital

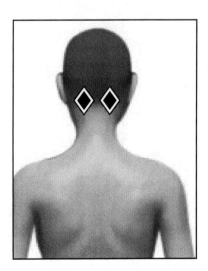

FLU 135
Cervical 1 - Sternocleidomastoid

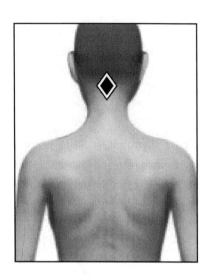 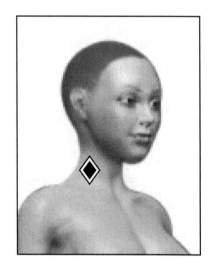

GUILLAIN BARRE OR POLYRADICULONEUROPATHY
Pineal - Oblongata

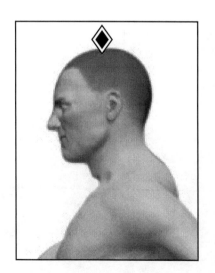 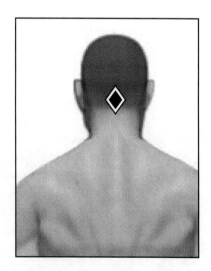

HANTAVIRUS
Mole - Kidney (ipsilateral)

* Note:
Check wherever there is a mole.

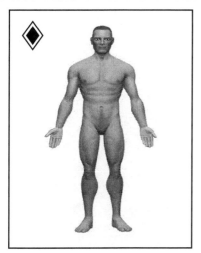
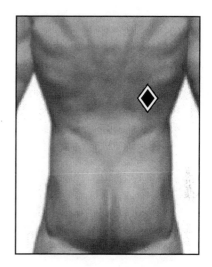

HANTAVIRUS
Pylorus - Anus

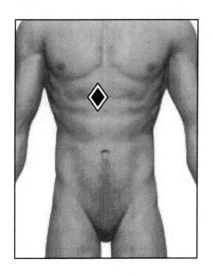
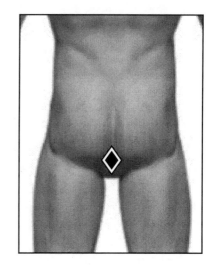

HEMORRHAGIC DENGUE
Oblongata - Bladder

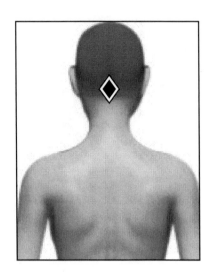
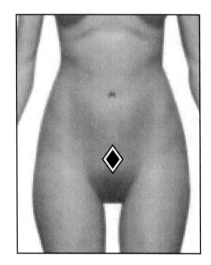

HEPATITIS B
Pleura (Right) - Liver

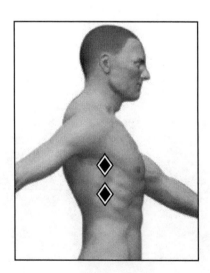

HERPE 5
Renal Calyx - Ureter

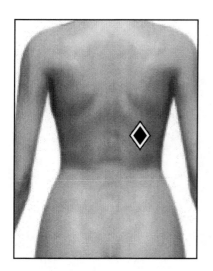 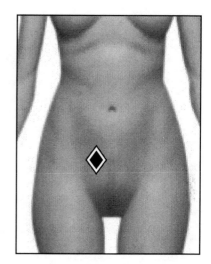

HERPES 1
Ascending Colon - Descending Colon

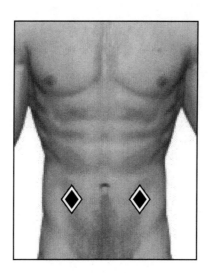

HERPES 2
Tonsil - Tonsil

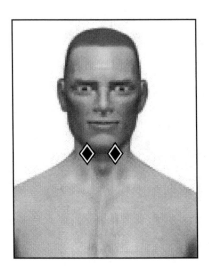

HERPES 3
Ulna - Ulna

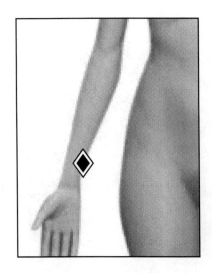 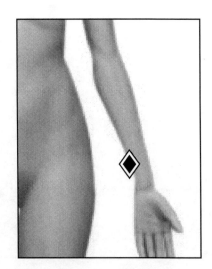

HERPES 4
Mouth (Corner) - Mouth (Corner)

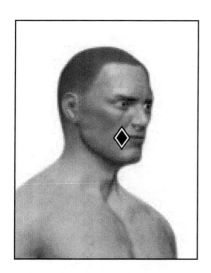 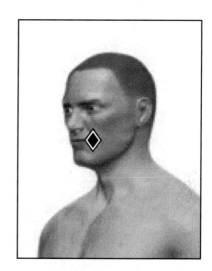

HERPES 6
Femoral Nerve - Femoral Nerve

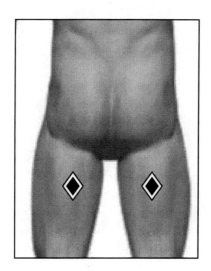

HERPES 7
Bladder - Sacrum

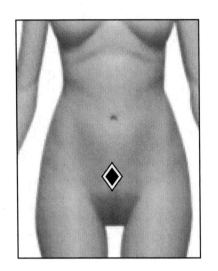
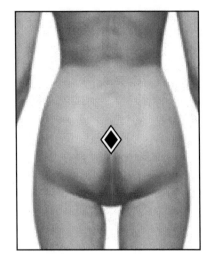

HIV
Adductor - Adductor

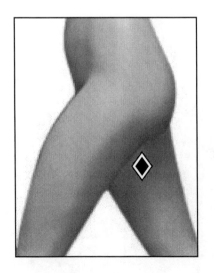
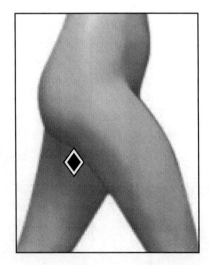

HIV
Rectum - Thymus

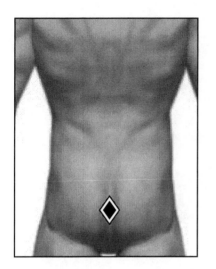 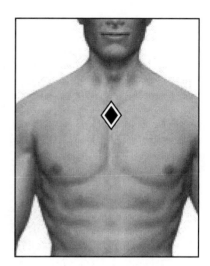

HIV 3
Groin Nerve - Groin Nerve

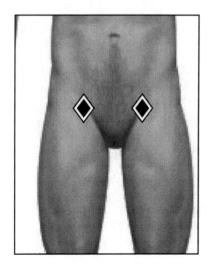

HIV 4
Lesser Trochanter - Lesser Trochanter

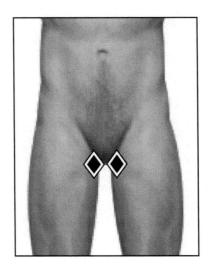

HTLV VIRUS
Suprapubic - Suprapubic

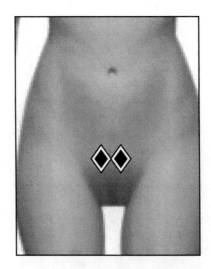

INFLUENZA
Trachea - Trachea

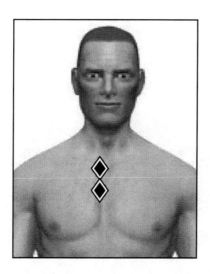

LEUKEMIA
Spleen - Duodenum

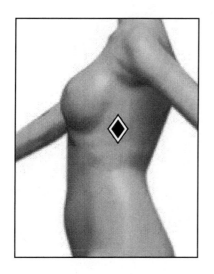
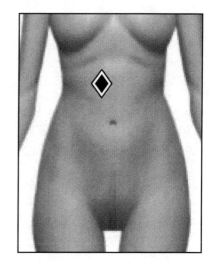

MEASLES
Stomach - Adrenals

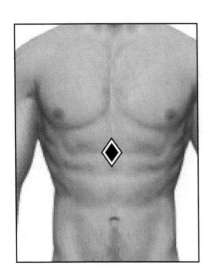
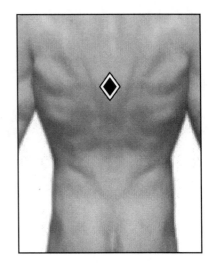

MENINGITIS
Thyroid - Oblongata

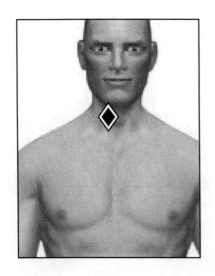
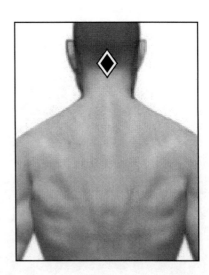

N1H1
Pancreatic Ligament - Spleen

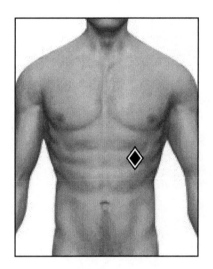 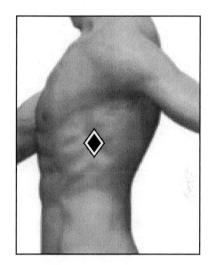

NEWCASTLE VIRUS
Cerebellum - Oblongata

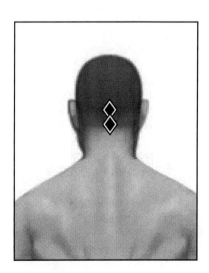

NORWALK
Douglas Pouch - Femoral Vein

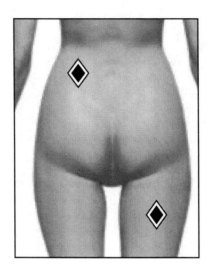

ORF VIRUS
Orbital Floor - Orbital Floor

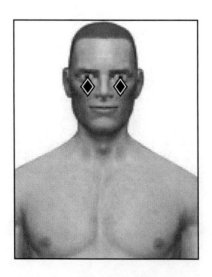

PAPILLOMAVIRUS
Prostate - Rectum

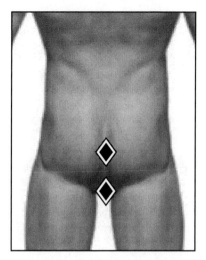

Prostate: Place magnet between anus and testicles

PAPILLOMAVIRUS
Anus - Anus

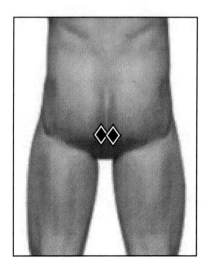

PARAMYXOVIRUS
Bladder Annex - Bladder Annex

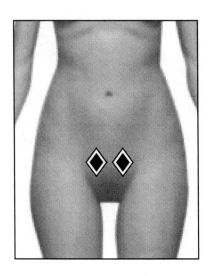

PARAMYXOVIRUS
Bladder Annex - Anus

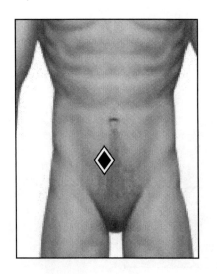
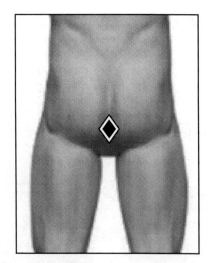

PAROTIDITIS OR MUMPS
Pudendal Nerve - Pudendal Nerve

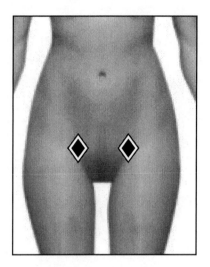

PARVOVIRUS
Fallopian - Fallopian

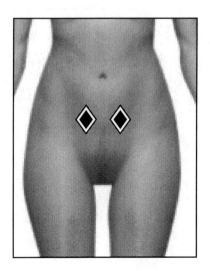

POLIOMYELITIS
Sciatic - Sciatic

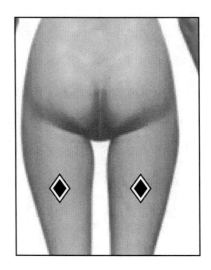

POLYOMA VIRUS
Temporal (Left) - Temporal (Left)

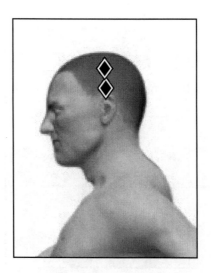

R-40 Virus
Sigmoid - Rectum

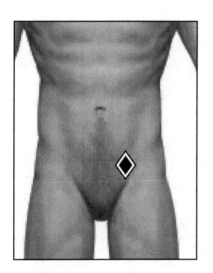 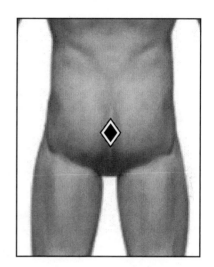

Rabies
Armpit - Armpit

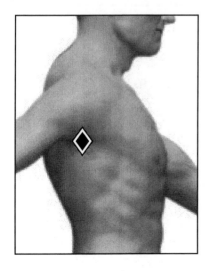 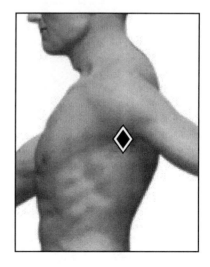

RABIES
Peripancreatic - Peripancreatic

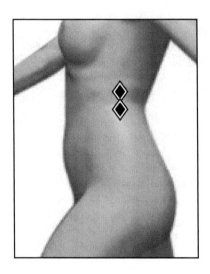

REOVIRUS
Circle of Willis - Circle of Willis

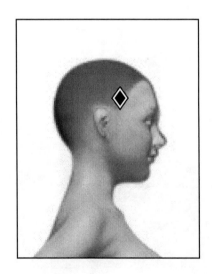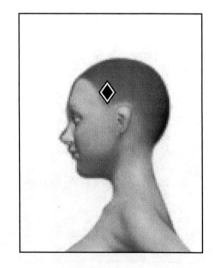

RESPIRATORY SYNCYTIAL VIRUS
Eyebrow - Eyebrow

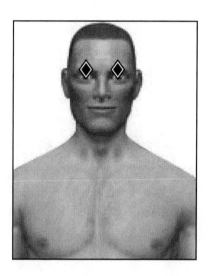

ROSEOLA
Groin Nerve - Liver

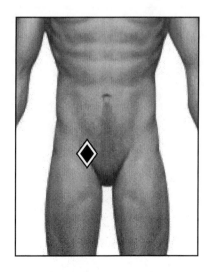
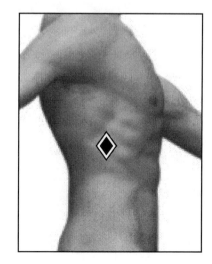

ROTAVIRUS
Coccyx - Coccyx

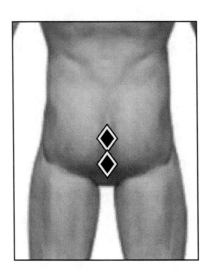

RUBEOLA (MEASLES)
Thymus - Parietal

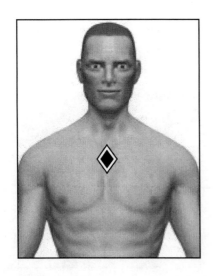 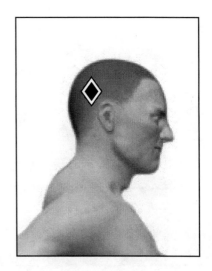

SMALLPOX
Appendix - Tongue

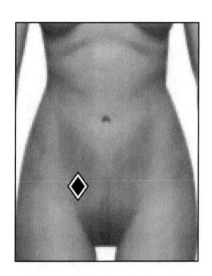 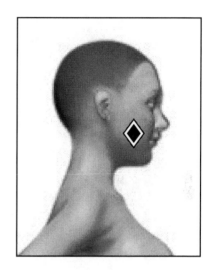

THYPHUS EXANTHEMATICUS
Temporal - Temporal

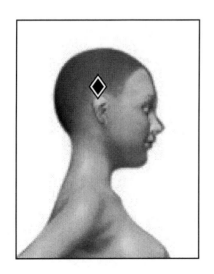 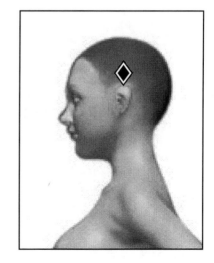

VACCINIA
Appendix - Femoral Vein

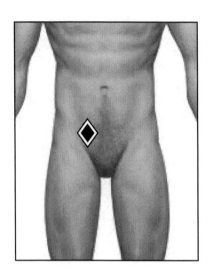 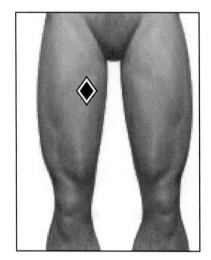

VARICELA (CHICKENPOX)
Ureter - Ureter

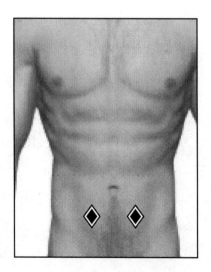

VHS
Vas Deferens - Larynx

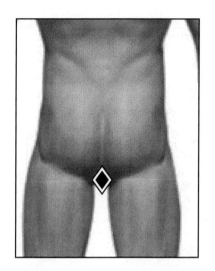 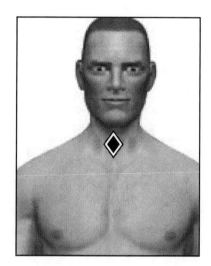

VIRAL ENCEPHALITIS
Parietal - Parietal

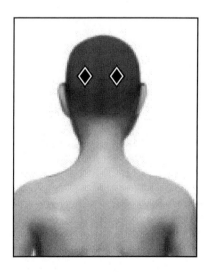

PLEURITIS
Infra Armpit - Infra Armpit

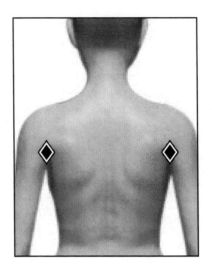

PLEURITIS
Pleura (Right) - Pleura (Left)

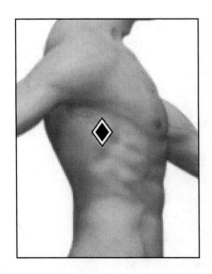 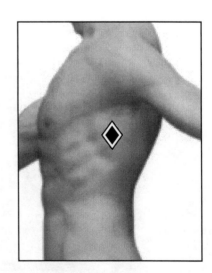

SINUSITIS
Frontal Sinus - Frontal Sinus

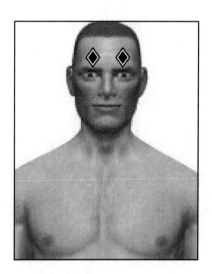

SINUSITIS
Paranasal - Paranasal

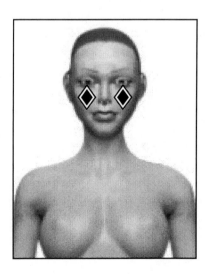

WARTS
Retro Tensor - Pectoral

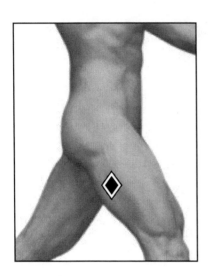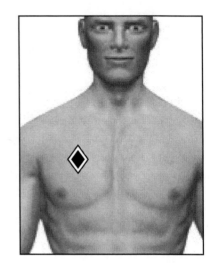

ZIKA
Costal - Descending Colon

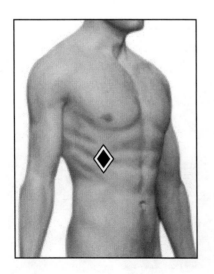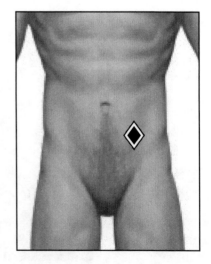

BACTERIAL INFECTION PAIRS

AEROBACTER AERUGINOSA
Pre-Frontal Pole - Pre-Frontal Pole

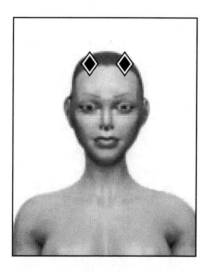

ANTHRAX
Cranial - Cranial

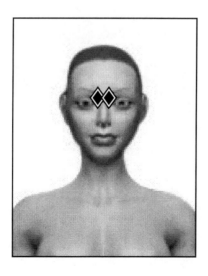

ATIPIC ESCHERICHIA COLI
Index - Index

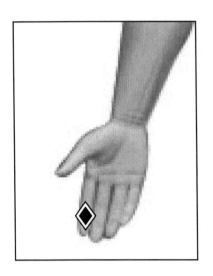 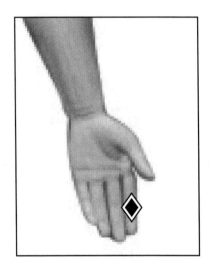

BORDETELLA PERTUSSIS
Contra Cecum - Contra Cecum

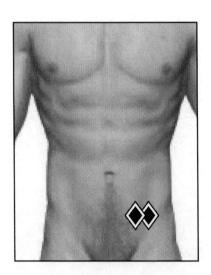

BORDETELLA PERTUSSIS
Larynx - Larynx

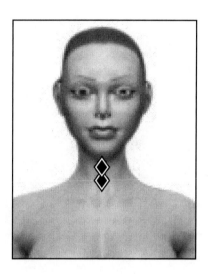

BORRELIA
Costal Hepatic - Costal Hepatic

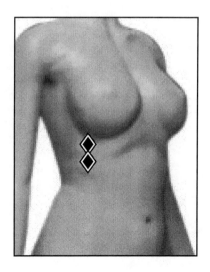

BOVINE TUBERCULOSIS
Perirenal - Perirenal

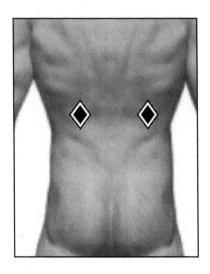

BRUCELLA ABORTUS
Diaphragm - Kidney (Ipsilateral)

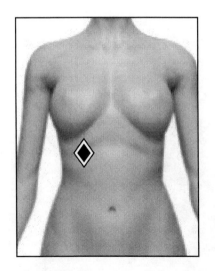 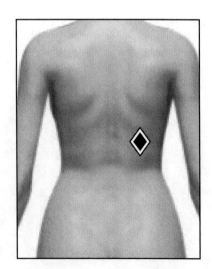

BRUCELLOSIS
Spleen - Liver

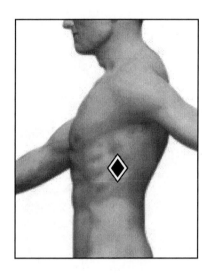 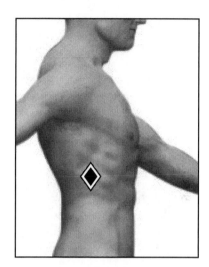

BURKHOLDERIA
Ascending Colon - Sacrum

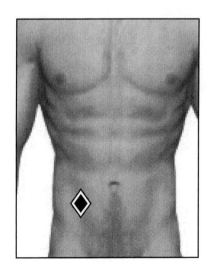 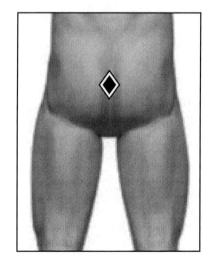

CAMPYLOBACTER JEJUNI
Sigmoid - Testicle

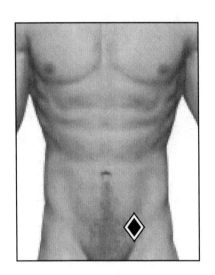
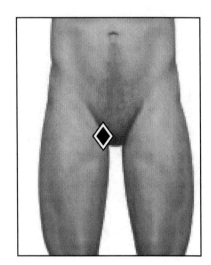

CHLAMYDIA PNEUMONIAE
Hip - Hip

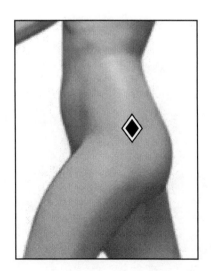
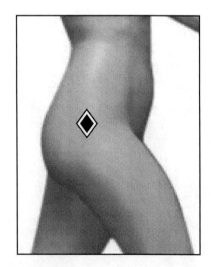

CHLAMYDIA TOUCANS AFRICANA
Stomach - Transverse Colon

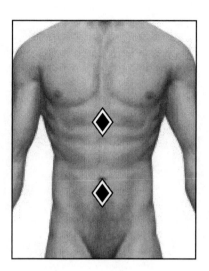

CHLAMYDIA TRACHOMATIS
Duodenum - Kidney (Left)

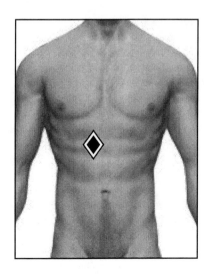 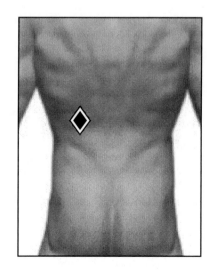

CHLAMYDIA TRACHOMATIS
Duodenum - Liver

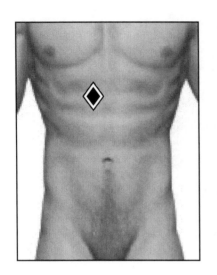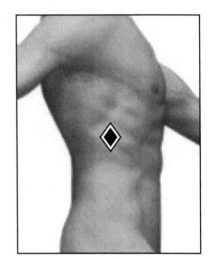

CLOSTRIDIUM BOTULINUM
Pancreas Tail - Liver

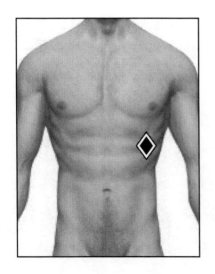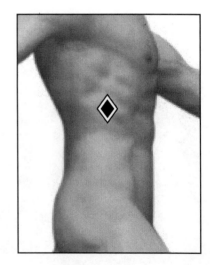

CLOSTRIDIUM DIFFICILE
Pancreas Head - Pylorus

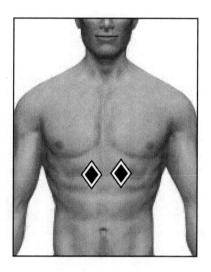

CLOSTRIDIUM MALIGNUM
Suprahepatic - Suprahepatic

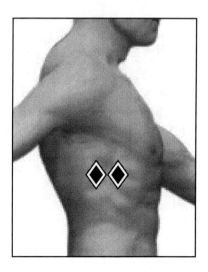

CLOSTRIDIUM PERFRINGENS
Esophagus - Pylorus

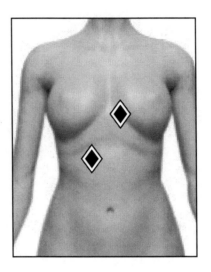

CLOSTRIDIUM PERFRINGENS
Stomach - Pylorus

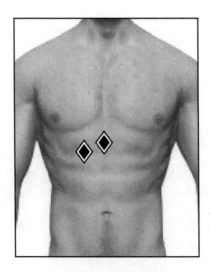

CLOSTRIDIUM TETANI
Kidney - Kidney

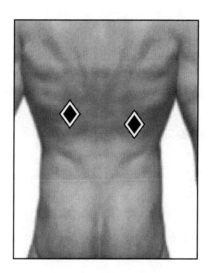

DIPHTHERIA
Subclavian - Subclavian

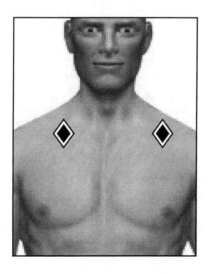

ENTEROBACTER CLOACAE
Descending Colon - Descending Colon

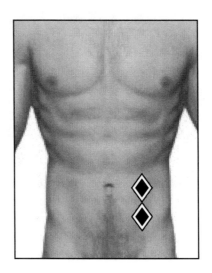

ENTEROBACTER PNEUMONIAE
Hiatus - Esophagus

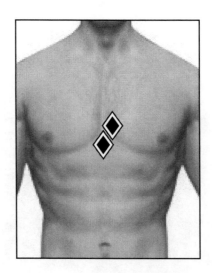

ENTEROBACTER PNEUMONIAE
Humerus - Humerus

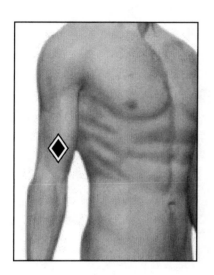
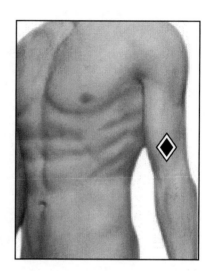

ENTEROCOCCUS
Bladder - Anus

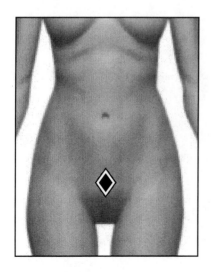
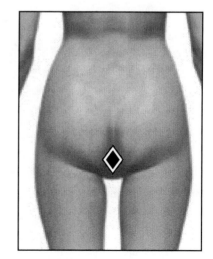

ENTEROCOCCUS
Lumbar Plexus - Lumbar Plexus

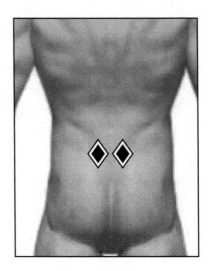

ESCHERICHIA COLI
Stomach - Thymus

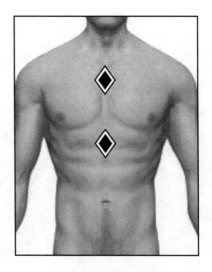

ESCHERICHIA COLI
Thymus - Liver

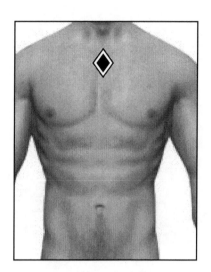 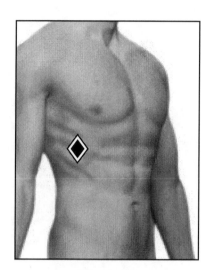

GARDNERELLA VAGINALIS
Tensor Fasciae Latae - Tensor Fasciae Latae

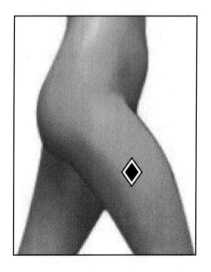 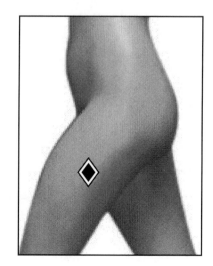

HELICOBACTER PYLORI
Hiatus - Testicle (Right)

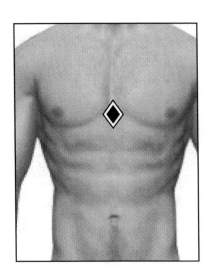 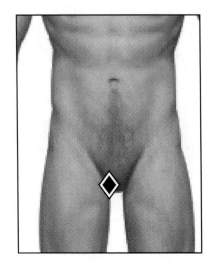

HIV
Thymus - Rectum

Note: Dr. Goiz believed that HIV was bacterial infection

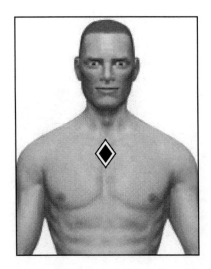 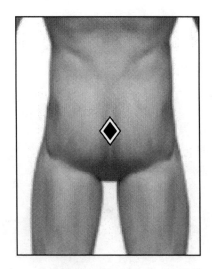

KLEBSIELLA NEUMONIAE
Lacrimal - Lacrimal

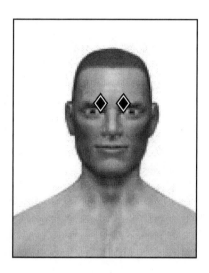

KLEBSIELLA PNEUMONIAE
Ascending Colon - Kidney (Right)

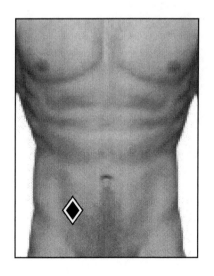 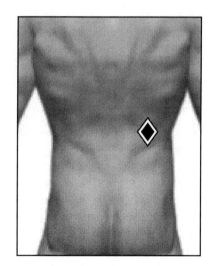

KLEBSIELLA PNEUMONIAE
Ascending Colon - Liver

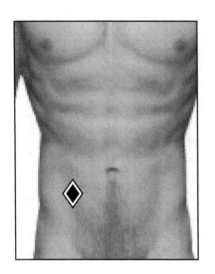 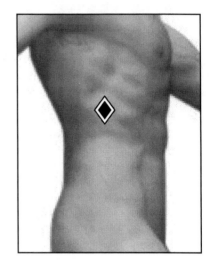

KLEBSIELLA PNEUMONIAE
Costal - Liver

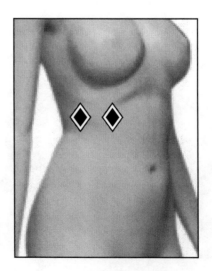

KLEBSIELLA PNEUMONIAE
Maxilla - Maxilla

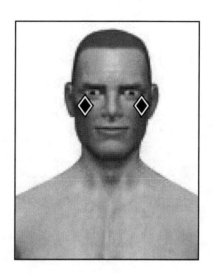

LEGIONELLA
Thoracic 2 - Thoracic 2

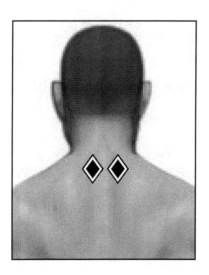

LEPROSY
Pancreatic Duct - Kidney (Right)

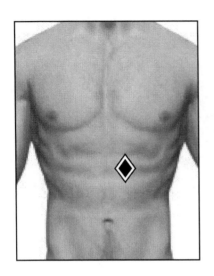 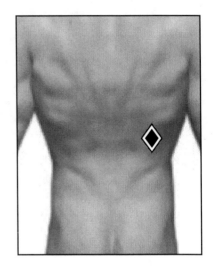

LISTERIA
Ascending Colon - Ascending Colon

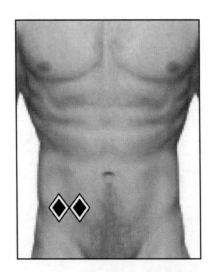

LISTERIA
Liver - Pylorus

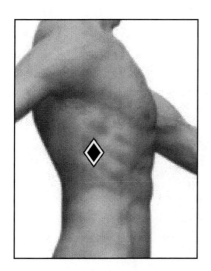
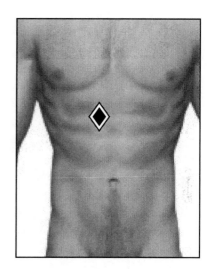

MENINGOCOCCUS
Thoracic - Lumbar

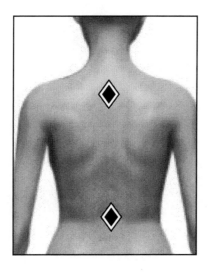

MORGANELLA TYPHUS
Perihepatic - Perihepatic

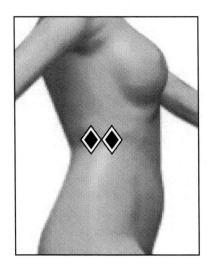

MYCOBACTERIUM LEPRAE
Scapula - Scapula

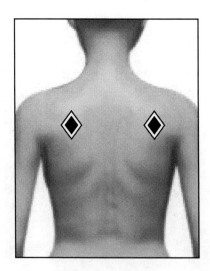

MYCOBACTERIUM TUBERCULOSIS
Supraspinatus - Supraspinatus

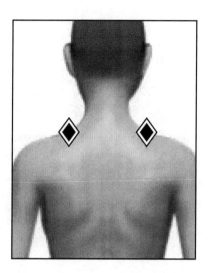

MYCOPLASMA TYPE 1
Temporo-Occipital - Temporo-Occipital

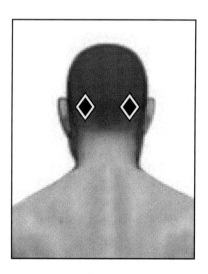

MYCOPLASMA TYPE 2
Pectoral - Pectoral

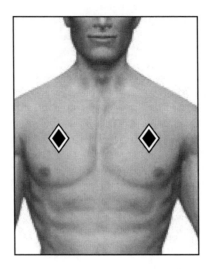

NEISSERIA CATARRHALIS
Eyelid - Eyelid

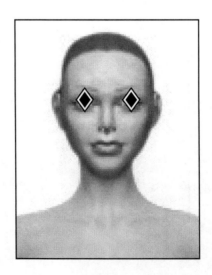

NEISSERIA CATARRHALIS
Greater Sciatic Notch - Greater Sciatic Notch

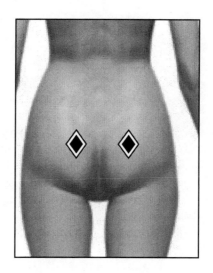

NEISSERIA GONORRHEA
Lumbar 4 - Lumbar 4

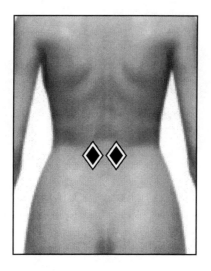

NEISSERIA GONORRHOEAE
Mandíbula - Mandíbula

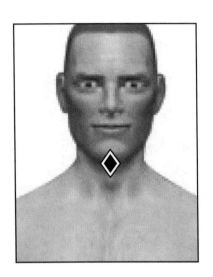
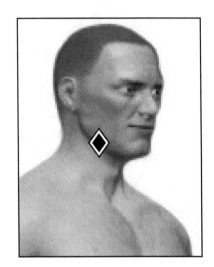

NOCARDIA AMERICANA
Preauricular - Preauricular

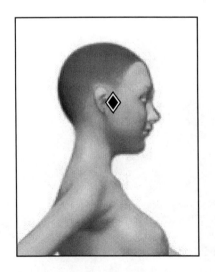
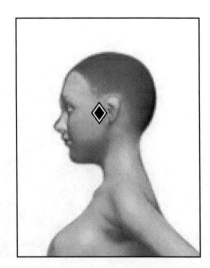

PARATYPHOID BACILLUS
Greater Trochanter - Kidney (Ipsilateral)

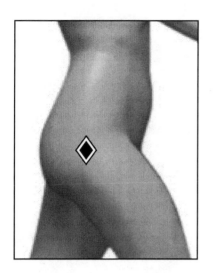
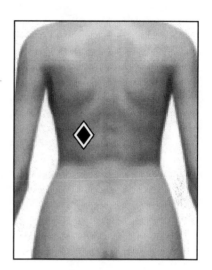

PASTEURELLA
Descending Colon - Kidney (Left)

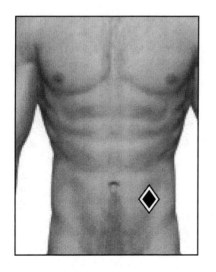
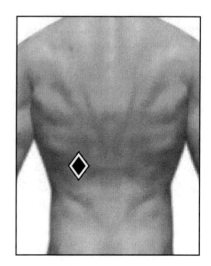

PASTEURELLA
Descending Colon - Liver

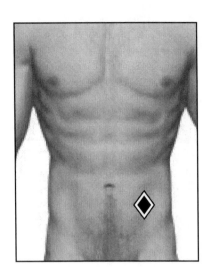
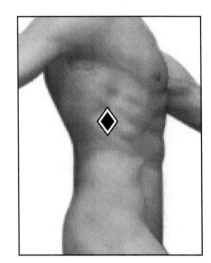

PASTEURELLA
Liver - Descending Colon

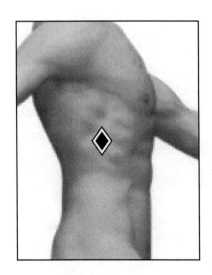
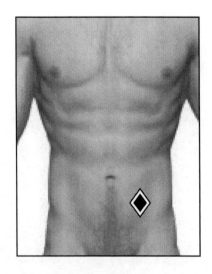

PNEUMOCOCCUS OR PNEUMONIA
Popliteal - Popliteal

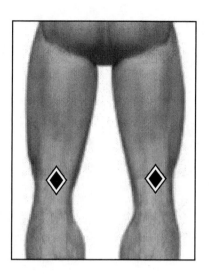

PROTEUS MIRABILIS
Costal - Costal

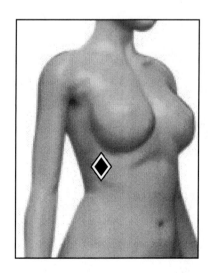 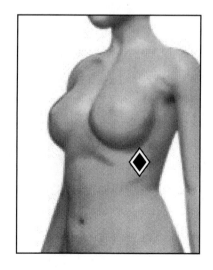

PROTEUS MIRABILIS
Fibula - Fibula

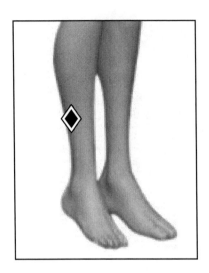 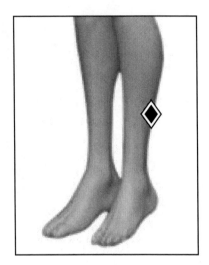

PROTEUS MIRABILIS
Mediastinum (Superior) - Mediastinum (Inferior)

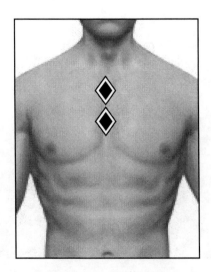

PROTEUS MIRABILIS
Renal Capsule - Renal Capsule

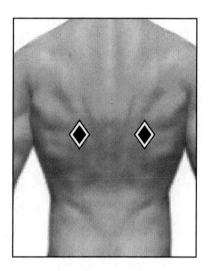

PROTEUS MIRABILIS
Sacrum - Sacrum

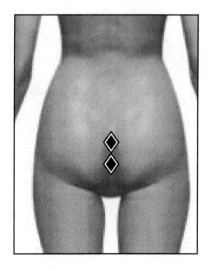

PROTEUS VULGARIS
Infra Chin - Infra Chin

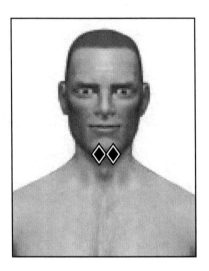

PSEUDOMONAS AERUGINOSA
Rectum - Rectum

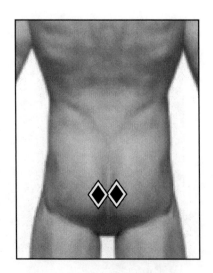

PSEUDOMONAS AEROGINOSA
Pleura - Pleura (Ipsilateral)

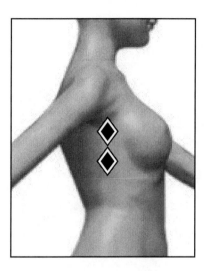

PSEUDOMONAS AERUGINOSA
Adrenal - Lung

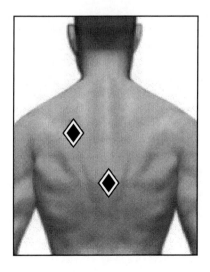

RICKETTSIA
Calcaneus - Calcaneus

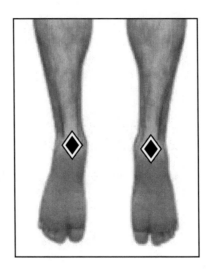

RICKETTSIA
Wrist - Wrist

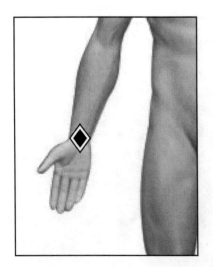 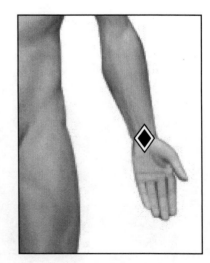

SALMONELLA TYPHI
Greater Trochanter - Greater Trochanter

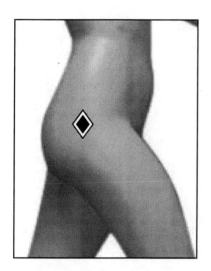 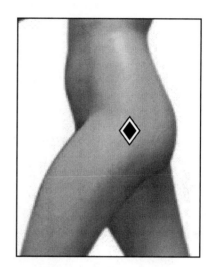

SHIGELLA
Achiles - Achiles

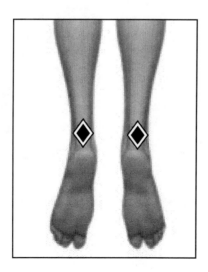

SPIROCHETE
Clitoris - Clitoris

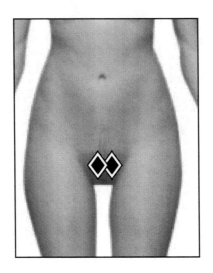

SPIROCHETE
Pancreatic Duct - Kidney (Left)

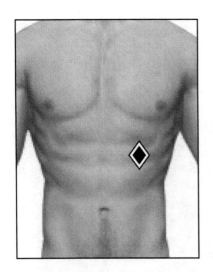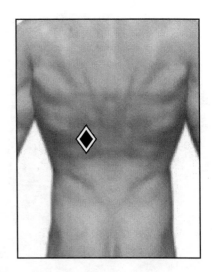

SPIROCHETE
Pancreatic Duct - Kidney (Right)

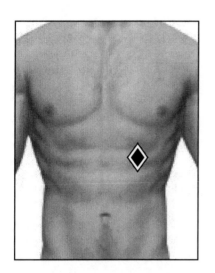
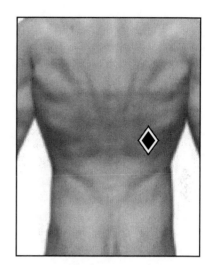

STAPHYLOCOCCUS ALBUS
Omentum - Omentum

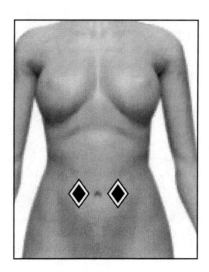

STAPHYLOCOCCUS AUREUS COAG NEG.
Pancreas Head - Adrenals

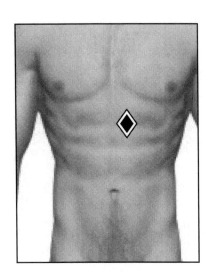 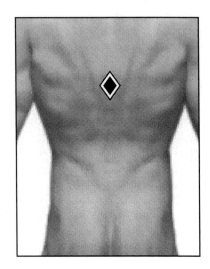

STAPHYLOCOCCUS AUREUS COAG. POS.
Pericardium - Pericardium

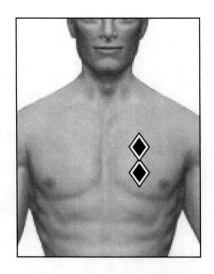

STAPHYLOCOCCUS AUREUS COAG. NEG.
Lumbar 5 - Lumbar 5

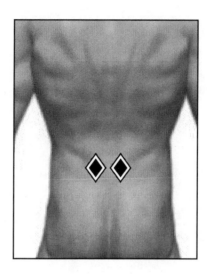

STAPHYLOCOCCUS AUREUS COAG. POS.
Appendix - Pleura

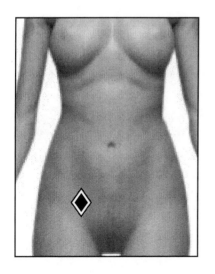
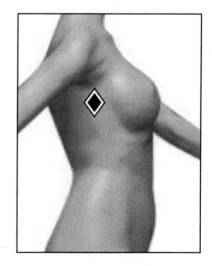

STAPHYLOCOCCUS AUREUS CUAG. POS.
Pleura - Appendix

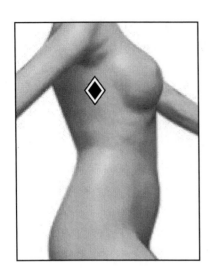 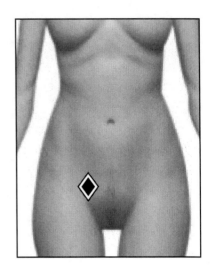

STAPHYLOCOCCUS AUREUS NEG.
Pancreas Head - Liver

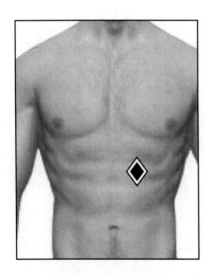 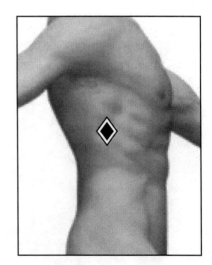

STAPHYLOCOCCUS EPIDERMIDIS
Mandibular Branch - Mandibular Branch

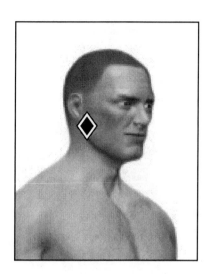 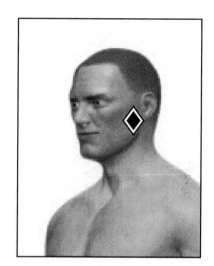

STREPTOCOCCUS A
Brachial - Brachial

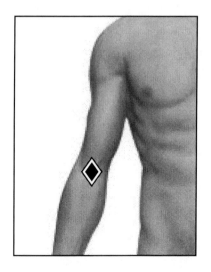 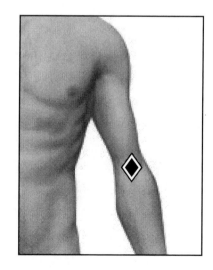

STREPTOCOCCUS A
Coronary Artery - Lung

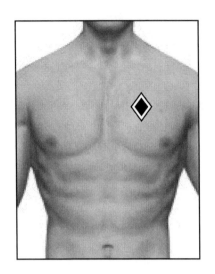 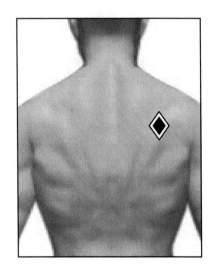

STREPTOCOCCUS AGALACTIAE
External Knee Ligament - Quadratus

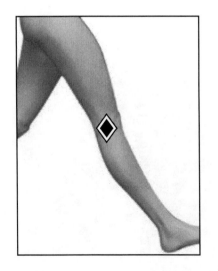 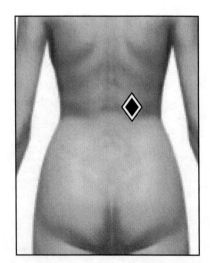

STREPTOCOCCUS B
Cardia - Adrenals

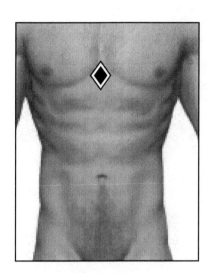
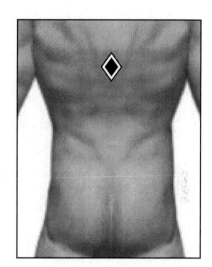

STREPTOCOCCUS BETA
Bursa - Elbow

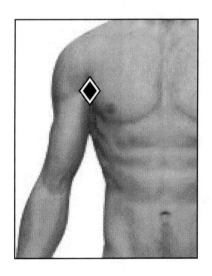
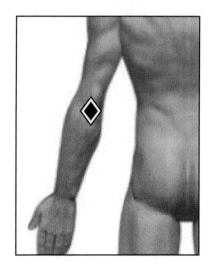

STREPTOCOCCUS C
Ischium (Ramus) - Ischium (Ramus)

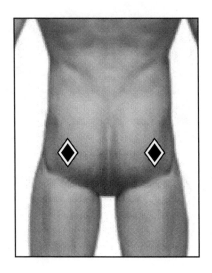

STREPTOCOCCUS C
Retroaxillary - Retroaxillary

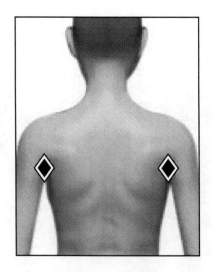

STREPTOCOCCUS FAECALIS
Cervical Plexus - Cervical Plexus

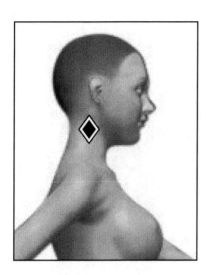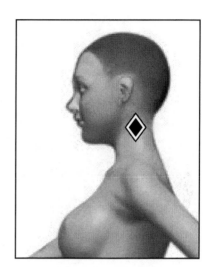

STREPTOCOCCUS FRAGILIS
Mandibular Angle - Mandibular Angle

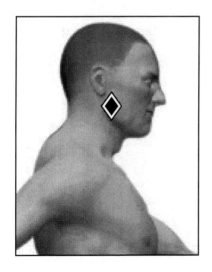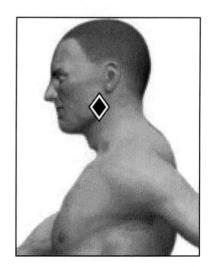

STREPTOCOCCUS G
Aortic Knob - Thoracic 7

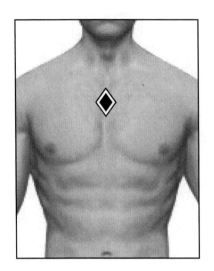 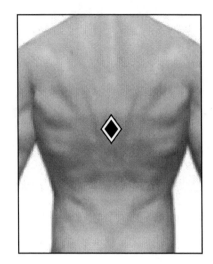

STREPTOCOCCUS G
Bladder - Bladder

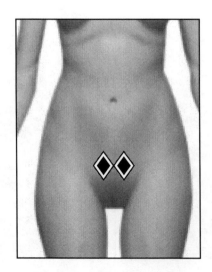

STREPTOCOCCUS G
Cardia - Pilorus

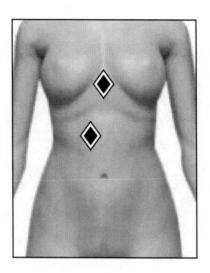

TREPONEMA BUCCALIS
Deltoid (Medial) - Deltoid (Medial)

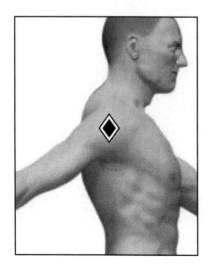 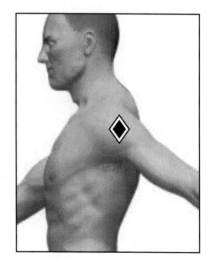

TREPONEMA PALLIDUM
Deltoid - Deltoid

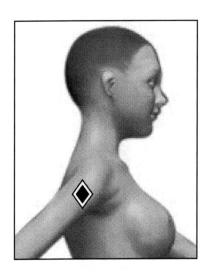 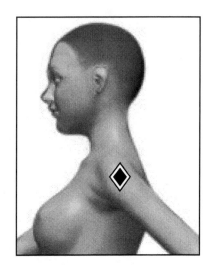

TREPONEMA PALLIDUM
Quadratus - Quadratus

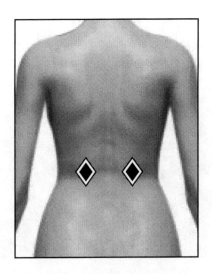

TRYPANOSOMA CRUZI
Costal Diaphragm - Costal Diaphragm

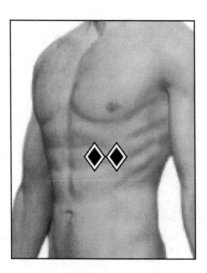

TRYPANOSOMA GAMBIE
Iliac Crest - Iliac Crest

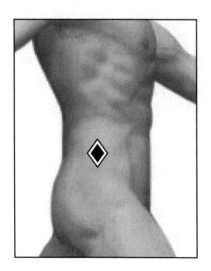 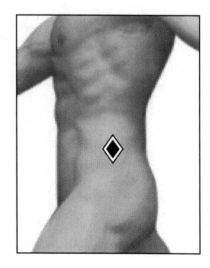

TUBERCULOSIS
Spermatic Duct - Spermatic Duct

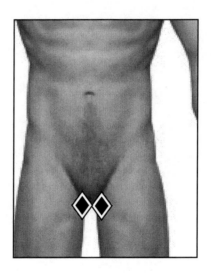

UREAPLASMA UREALYTICUM
Gluteo Minimus - Sacrum

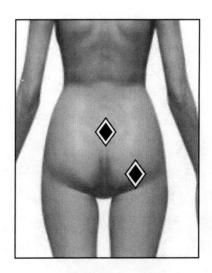

VEILLONELLA
Gluteus - Pylorus

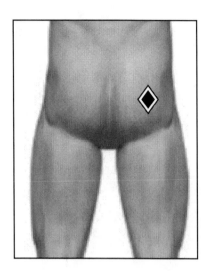 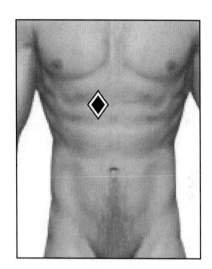

VIBRIO CHOLERAE
Transverse Colon - Bladder

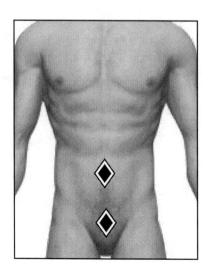

VIBRIO CHOLERAE
Transverse Colon - Liver

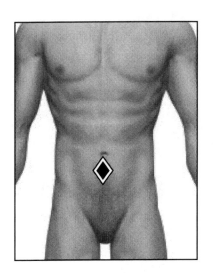 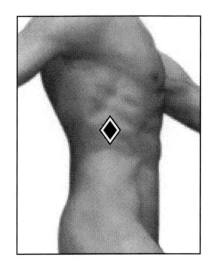

YELLOW FEVER
Pancreatic Ligament - Descending Colon

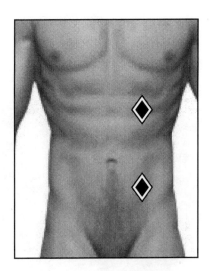

YERSINIA
Flank - Flank

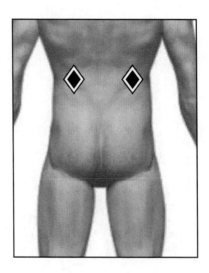

YERSINIA PESTIS
Vagina - Vagina

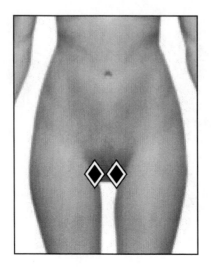

YERSINIA PESTIS
Testicle - Testicle

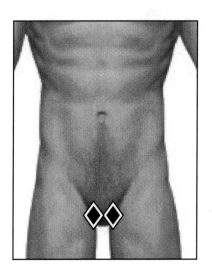

YERSINIA PESTIS
Vagina - Throat

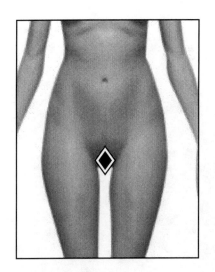 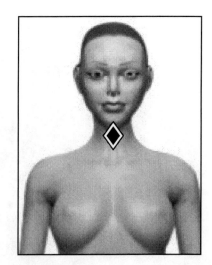

YERSINIA PESTIS OR SPLEEN DYSFUNCTION
Spleen - Spleen

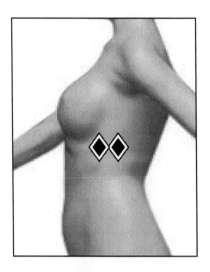

YERSINIA PNEUMONIAE
Latissimus - Latissimus

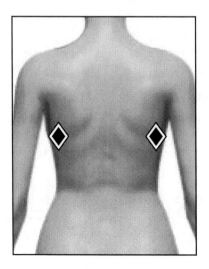

Mycotic (Fungal) Infection Pairs

Actinomyces
Bursa - Bursa

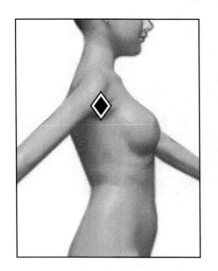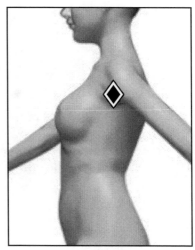

Aspergillus
Canthus - Canthus

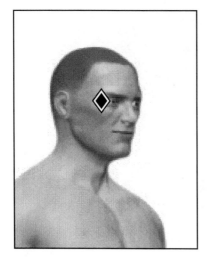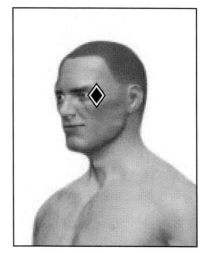

BLASTOMYCOSIS
Greater Trochanter - Tensor Fasciae Latae

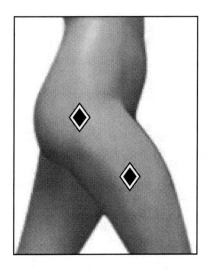

CANDIDA ALBICANS
Diaphragm - Diaphragm

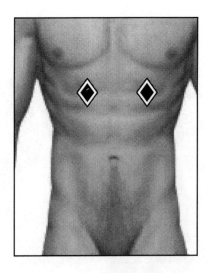

CRYPTOCOCCUS
Pre-Pineal - Bladder

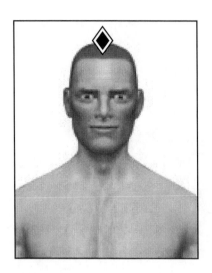 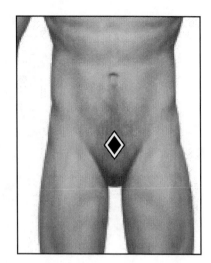

CRYPTOPHYTE
Post-Pineal - Bladder

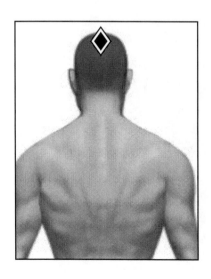 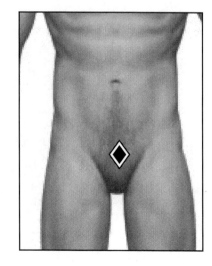

HISTOPLASMA CAPSULATUM
Esophagus - Bladder (Left)

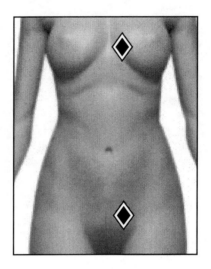

INTESTINAL MYCELIA
Pylorus - Ureter

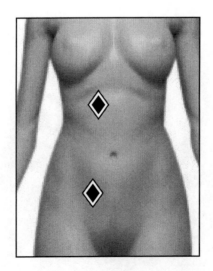

MALASSEZIA FURFUR
Tibia - Tibia

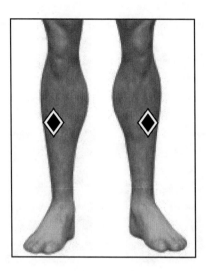

MICROSPORUM
Knee (Internal Ligament) - Internal Malleolus

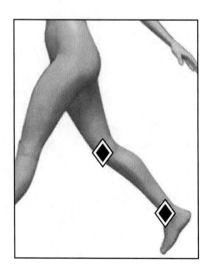

MICROSPORUM
Radius - Radius

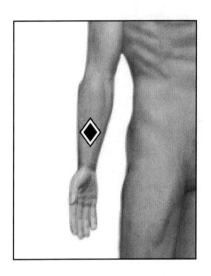
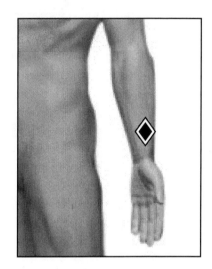

PNEUMOCYSTIS CARINII
Chondral - Chondral

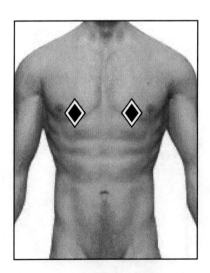

TRICHOPHYTON
Vena Cava - Vena Cava

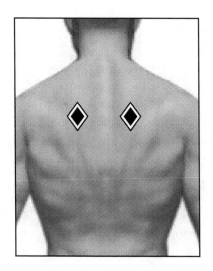

TRICHOPHYTON
Rib 1 - Rib 1

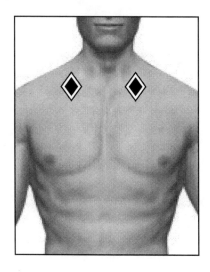

YEAST
Anus - Pylorus

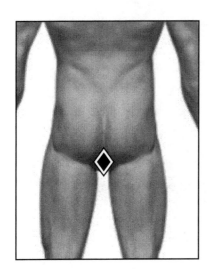 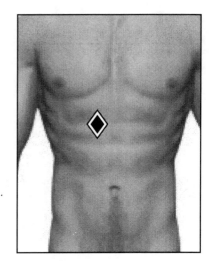

PARASITIC INFECTION PAIRS

AMEBIASIS
Pylorus - Kidney (Left)

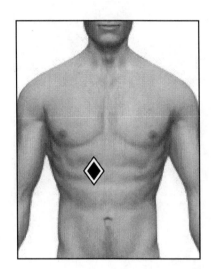
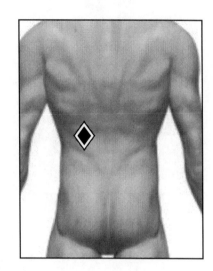

BABESIA
Gluteus - Femoral

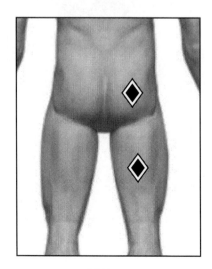

BALANTIDIUM TYPHUS
Cervical - Deltoid

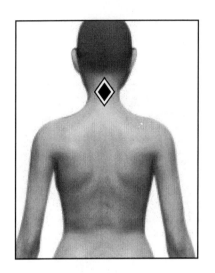 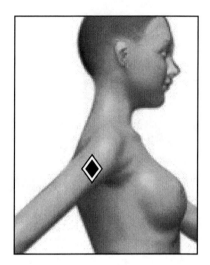

BALANTIDIUM TYPHUS
Cervical 3 - Supraspinatus

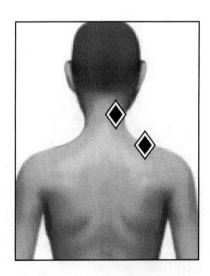

BLASTOCYSTIS HOMINIS
Neck - Neck

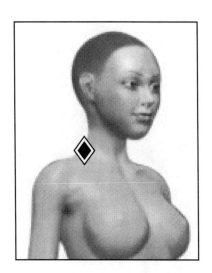 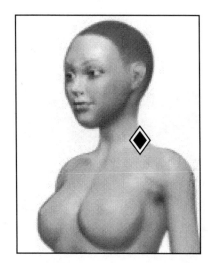

CISTICERCOSIS
Subdiaphragm - Subdiaphragm

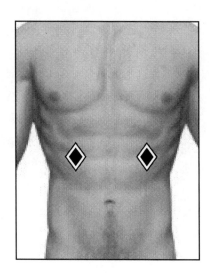

ECHINOCOCCUS GRANULOSUS
Pancreas - Spleen

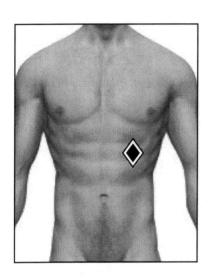 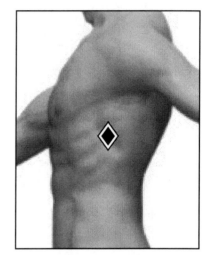

ENTAMOEBA HISTOLYTICA
Parietal - Transverse Colon

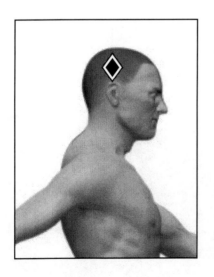 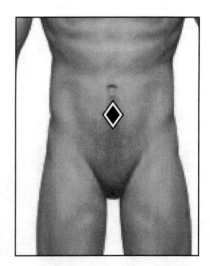

FASCIOLOSIS BURSKI
Esophagus - Esophagus

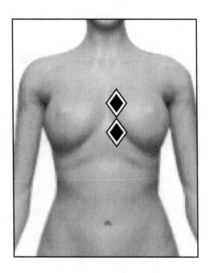

FILARIA
Mastoid - Mastoid

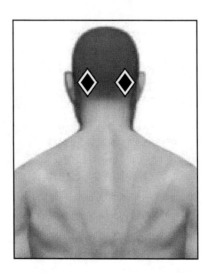

GIARDIA LAMBLIA
Diaphragmatic Hiatus - Diaphragmatic Hiatus

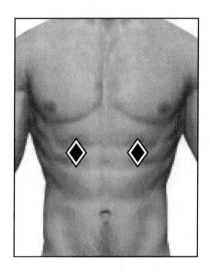

GIARDIA LAMBLIA
Epigastrium - Epigastrium

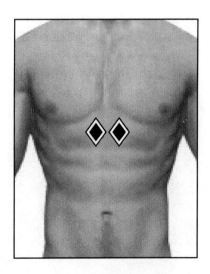

GIARDIA LAMBLIA
Transverse Colon - Colon Descending

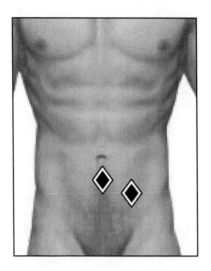

HEPATIC ABSCESS AMOEBA
Liver - Kidney (Left)

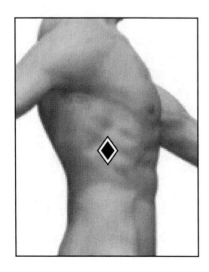 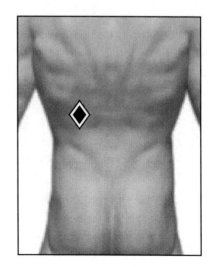

INTESTINAL PARASITE
Gluteus - Gluteus

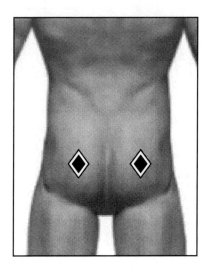

LEISHMANIASIS
Deltoid - Kidney

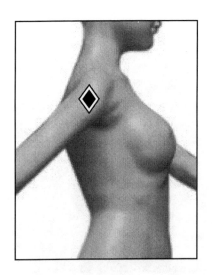 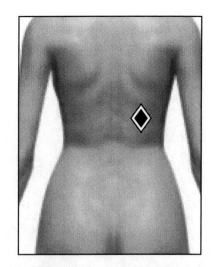

LEPTOSPIRA
Adrenal - Rectum

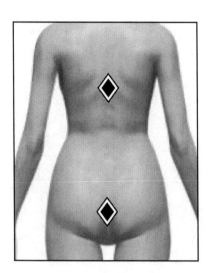

MALARIA
Cheekbone - Kidney (Contralateral)

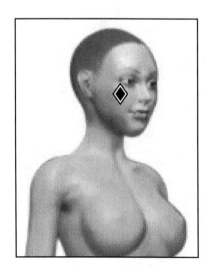 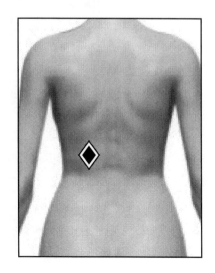

MALARIA
Palm - Palm

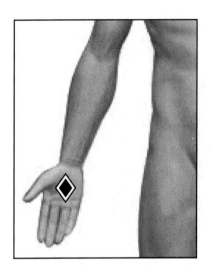
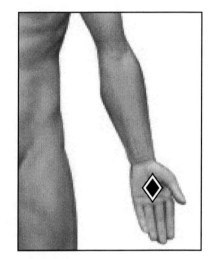

ONCHOCERCIASIS
Ischium - Ischium

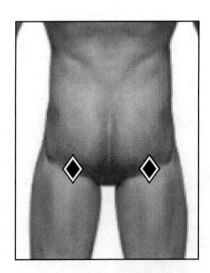

PINWORM
Pylorus - Liver

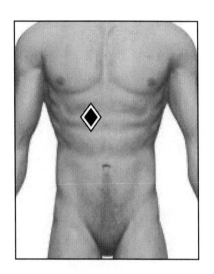
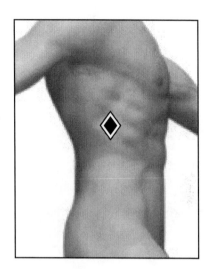

PLASMODIUM FALCIPARUM
Cervical 1 - Pylorus

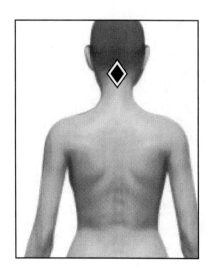
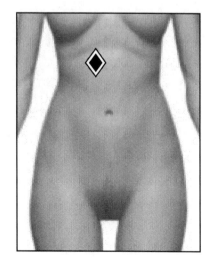

SCABIES OR MANGE
Tongue - Tongue

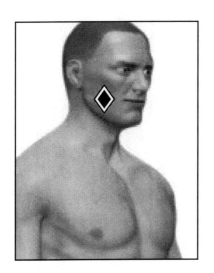 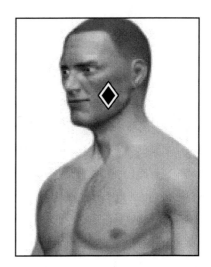

SCHISTOSOMA
Colon (Descending) - Quadriceps

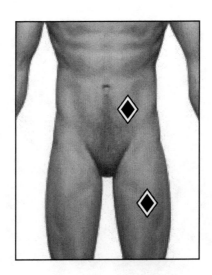

TOXOCARIASIS
Liver (Posterior Lobe) - Kidney (Ipsilateral)

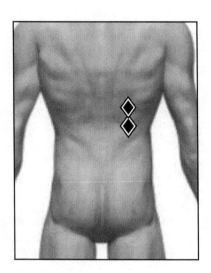

TOXOCARIASIS
Retrohepatic - Retrohepatic

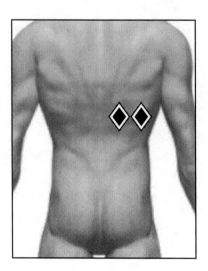

TOXOPLASMOSIS
Ear (Over Canal) - Ear (Over Canal)

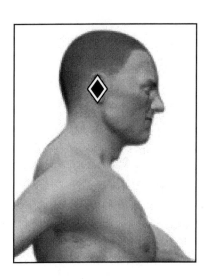 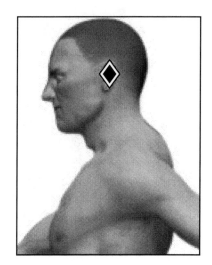

TRICHINOSIS
Hiatus - Tongue

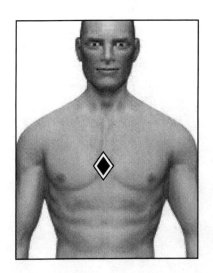 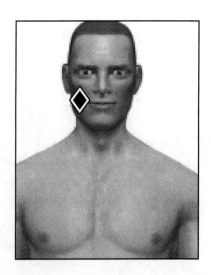

TRICHINELLA SPIRALIS
Pylorus - Tongue

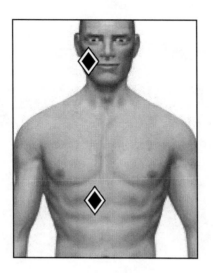

TRICHOMONIASIS
Cecum - Cecum

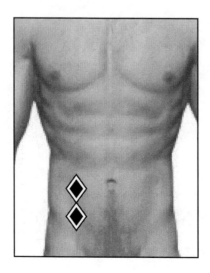

TRICHOMONIASIS
Cecum - Kidney (Right)

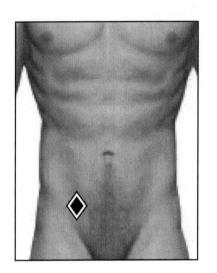 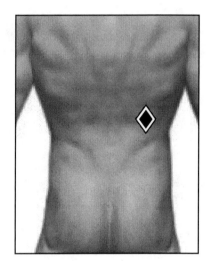

TRICHOMONIASIS
Ileocecal Valve - Kidney (Right)

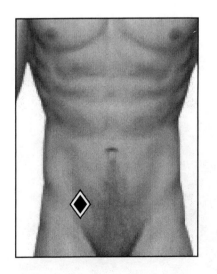 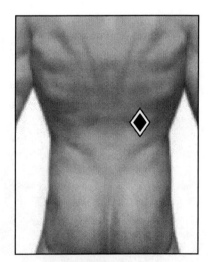

DYSFUNCTIONAL PAIRS (ORGANS/GLANDS)

ADRENAL DYSFUNCTION
Adrenal - Adrenal

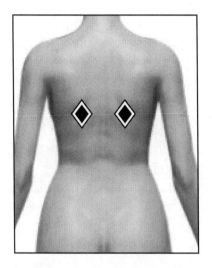

ALLERGIC ASTHMA
Adrenals - All Anterior

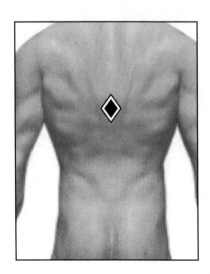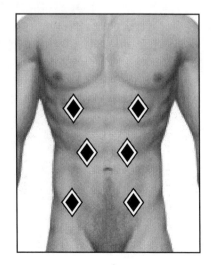

PARASYMPATHETIC DYSFUNCTION
Cervical - Sacrum

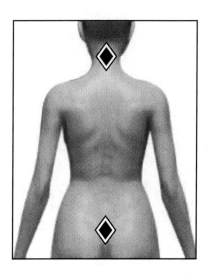

DUODENAL DYSFUNCTION
Duodenum - Duodenum

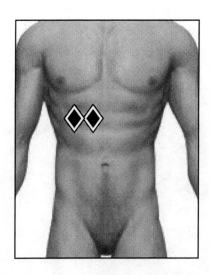

DIABETES MELLITUS
Duodenum - Kidney (Right)

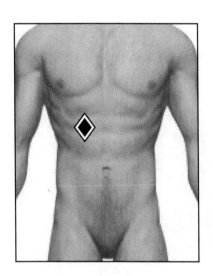 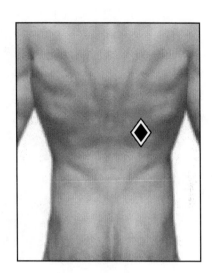

MONOARTICULAR ARTHRITIS
Groin Nerve - Joints

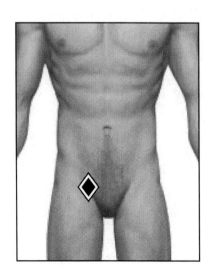 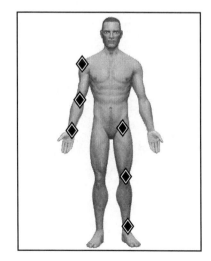

INTESTINAL DYSFUNCTION
Kidney - Sacrum (Contralateral)

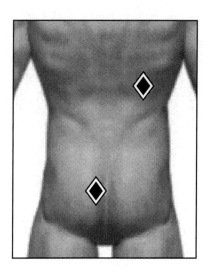

CIRRHOSIS
Liver - Kidney (Right)

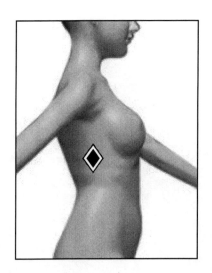 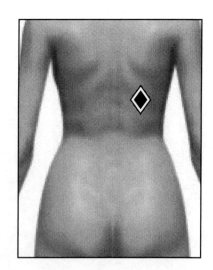

OVARIAN DYSFUNCTION
Ovary - Ovary

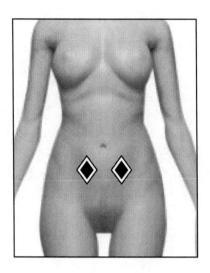

GLANDULAR DYSFUNCTION
Parathyroid - Parathyroid

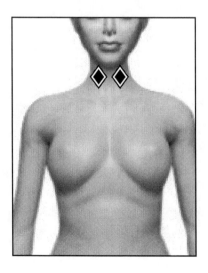

VITILIGO OR HYPOCHROMIA
Pineal - Pineal

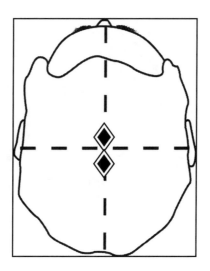

DIABETES INSIPIDUS
Pituitary - Oblongata

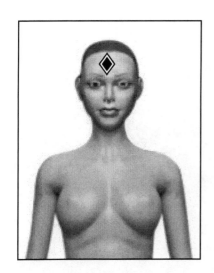 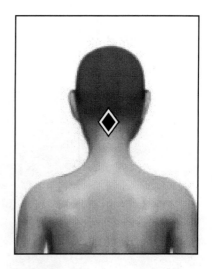

PITUITARY DYSFUNCTION
Pituitary - Pituitary

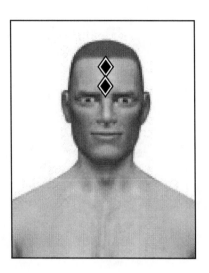

PROSTATE DYSFUNCTION
Prostate - Prostate

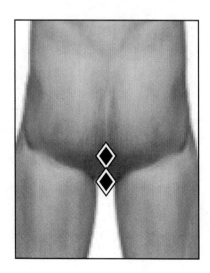

PYLORUS DYSFUNCTION
Pylorus - Pylorus

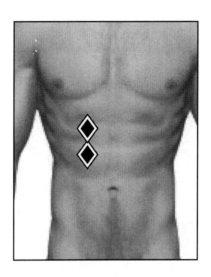

SYMPATHETIC NERVOUS DYSFUNCTION
Sternocleidomastoid - Sternocleidomastoid

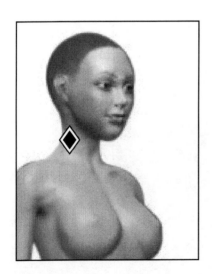 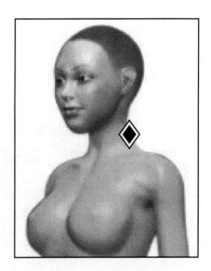

STOMACH DYSFUNCION
Stomach - Stomach

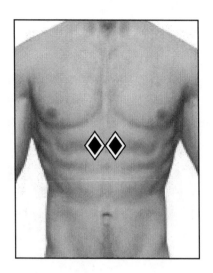

THYMUS DYSFUNCTION
Thymus - Thymus

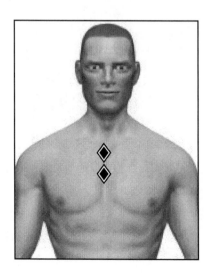

THYROID DYSFUNCTION
Thyroid - Thyroid

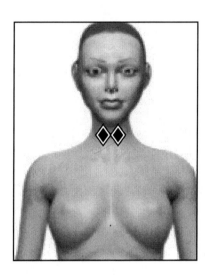

COLON DYSFUNCTION
Transverse Colon - Transverse Colon

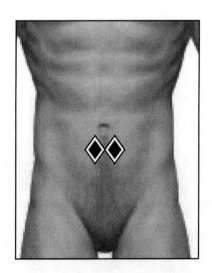

TOXINS (DETOXIFICATION) PAIRS

HEPATITIS C
Liver - Liver

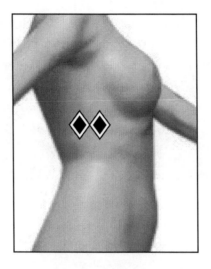

DETOXIFICATION TOXINS
Liver (Posterior Lobe) - Kidney (Left)

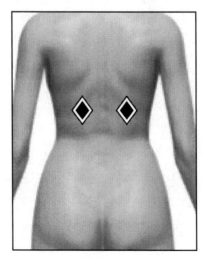

RENAL TOXINS
Renal Capsule - Bladder

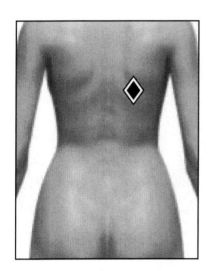 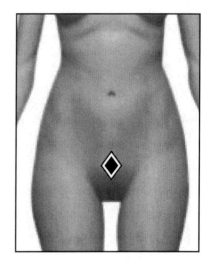

TOXOIDS
Nose - Nose

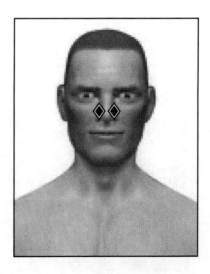

Reservoirs Pairs

Bacteria Reservoir
Spleen - Lung

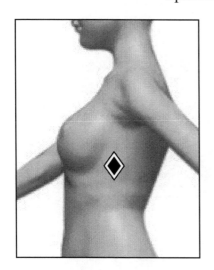
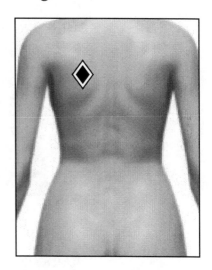

Bacteria Reservoir
Pleura (Right) - Peritoneum

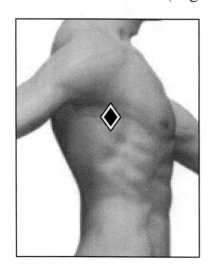
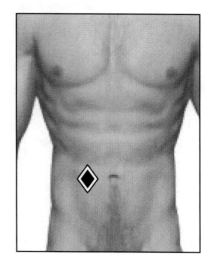

HIV RESERVOIR
Renal Capsule - Kidney (Ipsilateral)

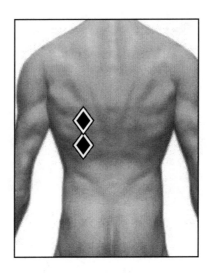

PARASITE RESERVOIR
Interiliac - Sacrum

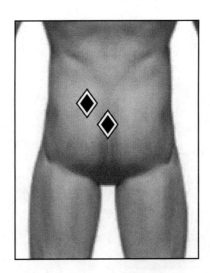

PARASITE RESERVOIR
Interiliac - Interiliac

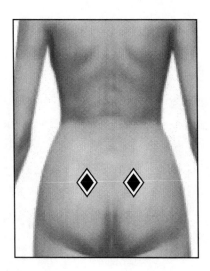

PARASITE RESERVOIR
Interiliac - Kidney

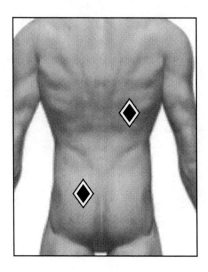

PRIONS RESERVOIR
Cardia - Temporal (Right)

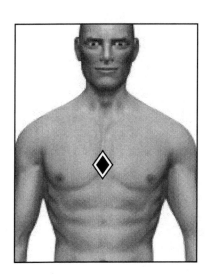
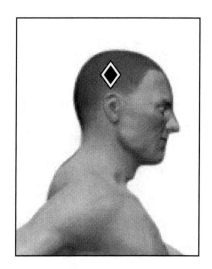

RABIES RESERVOIR
Bite - Armpit

Note: place magnet wherever the bite is.

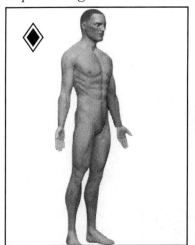
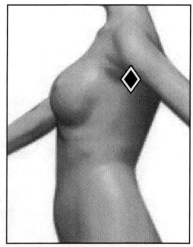

TUBERCULOSIS RESERVOIR
Callosum Edge - Callosum Edge

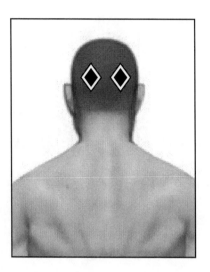

TUBERCULOSIS RESERVOIR
Head Fibula - Head Fibula

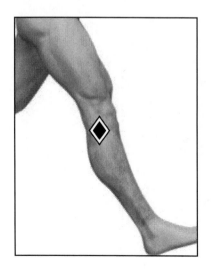 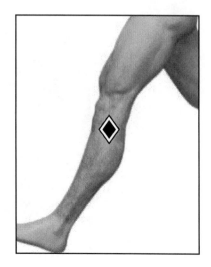

UNIVERSAL RESERVOIR
Pelvic Floor - Pelvic Floor

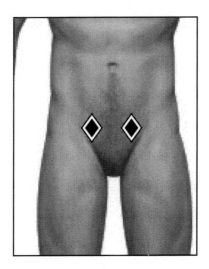

UNIVERSAL RESERVOIR
Subdiaphragmatic - Subdiaphragmatic

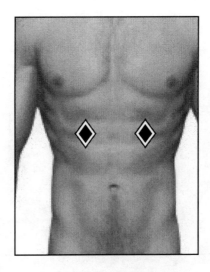

UNIVERSAL RESERVOIR
Teeth - Kidney (Ipsilateral)

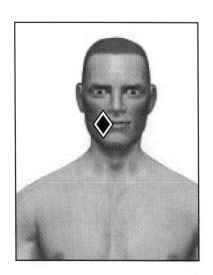
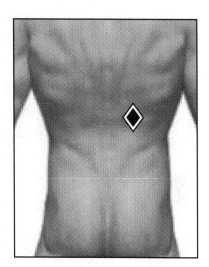

UNIVERSAL RESERVOIR
Vagus Nerve - Kidney (Contralateral)

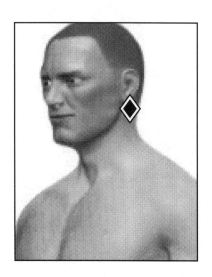
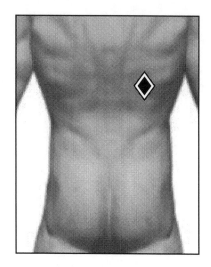

VIRUS RESERVOIR
Gallbladder - Gallbladder

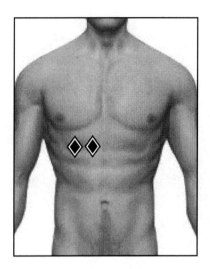

Emotional Pairs

Arrogance
Adrenal - Liver

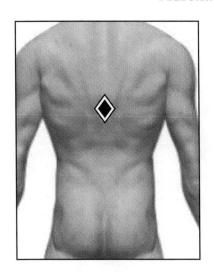
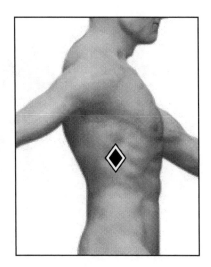

Character
Interciliar - Oblongata

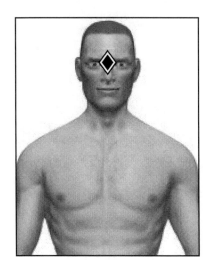
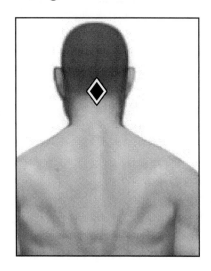

CRIMINALITY, AGGRESSIVENESS
Temporal (Right) - Temporal (Right)

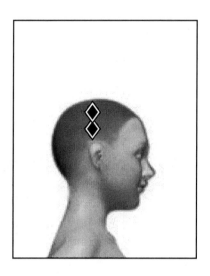

CRUELTY
Oblongata - Heart

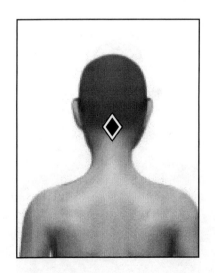 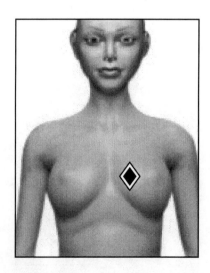

DOUBT
Back of Hands or Feet - Foot Instep

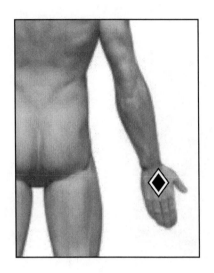
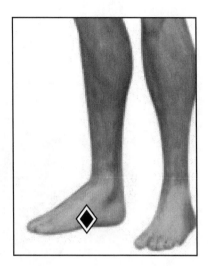

EEDIPUS COMPLEX
Belly Button - Uterus

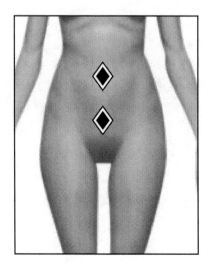

ELECTRA COMPLEX
Belly Button - Testicle

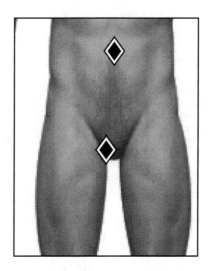

ENVY
Heart - Pancreas

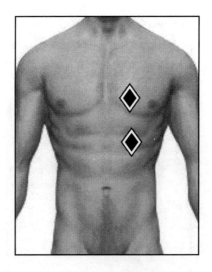

FEAR
Patella - Patella

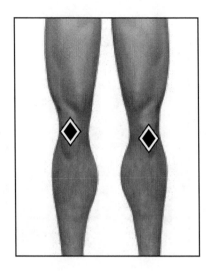

GLUTTONY
Stomach - Heart

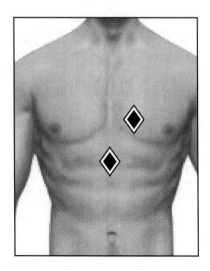

GREED
Thymus - Pituitary

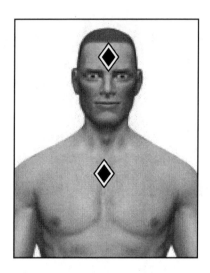

GUILT
Lung - Lung

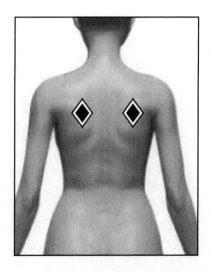

HATRED
Amygdala - Thymus

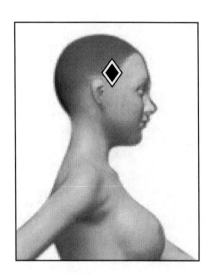 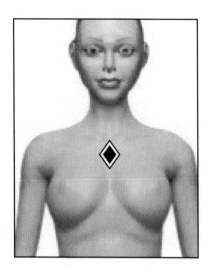

HAUGHTINESS
Median Fissure - Median Fissure

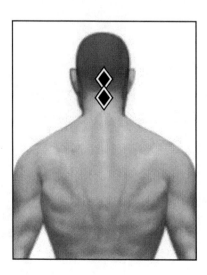

IMPATIENCE
Thymus - Ovary or Testicle

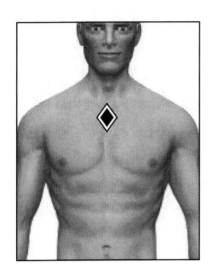 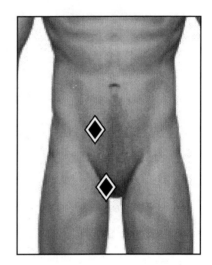

INSPIRATION (OVER THINKING)
Sylvian Fissure - Sylvian Fissure

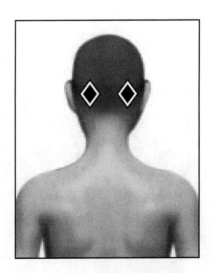

INTOLERANCE
Windpipe - Heart

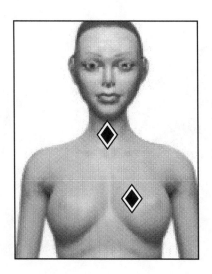

JELOUSY
Atlas - Uterus

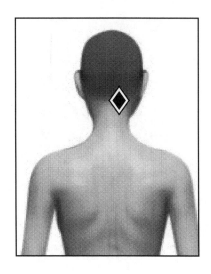
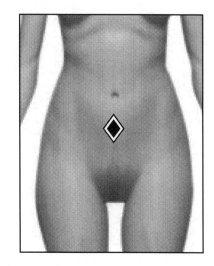

LAZINESS
Spleen - Hypothalamus

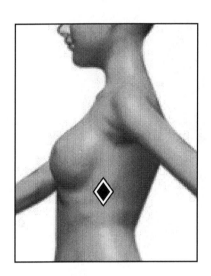
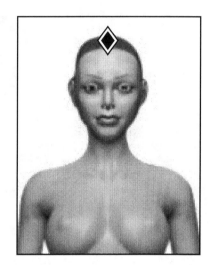

LUST
Pineal - Prostate or Uterus

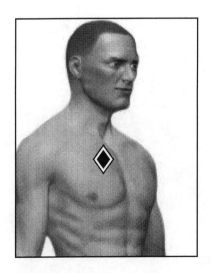
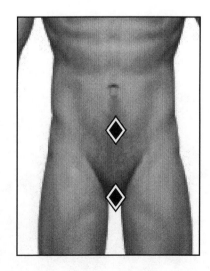

MALIGNITY
Occipital - Testicles or Vajina

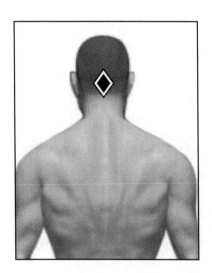 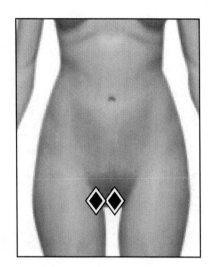

MATERIALISM
Transverse Colon - Testicle or Ovary

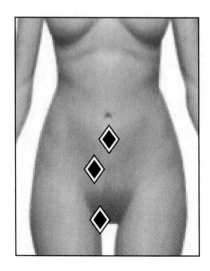

MYTHOMANIAC
Post-Pineal - Post-Pineal

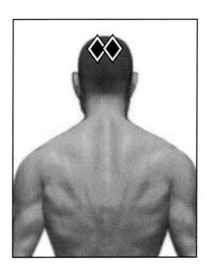

RAGE
Liver - Heart

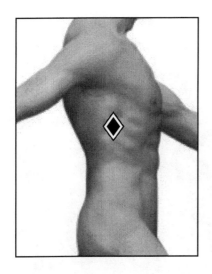 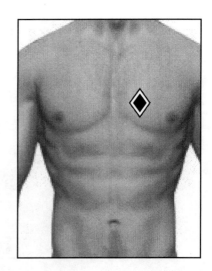

RESENTMENT
Heart - Bladder

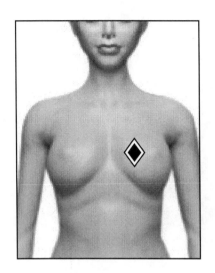
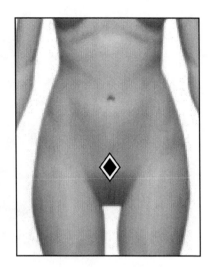

SADNESS
Lung - Heart

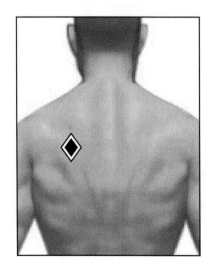
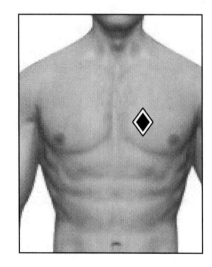

SADNESS
Lung - Oblongata

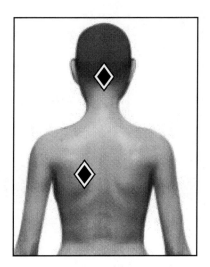

SPECIAL PAIRS

ARRHYTHMIA
Atrioventricular Sinus - Kidney

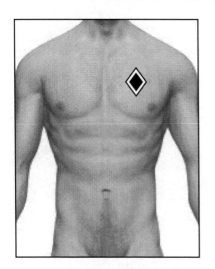 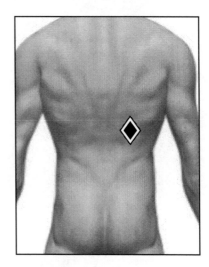

ATTENTION DEFICIT
Parietal - Kidney (Ipsilateral)

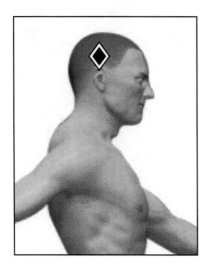 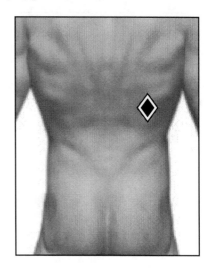

CEREBRAL MICROCIRCULATION, EMPHYSEMA, HYPERTENSION
Temple - Temple

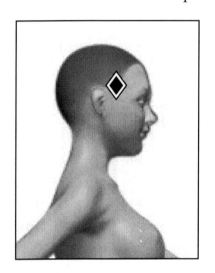
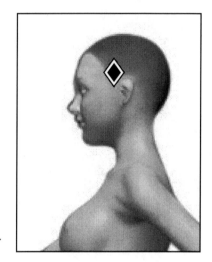

CHRONIC INTOXICATION
Palatine - Kidney (Ipsilateral)

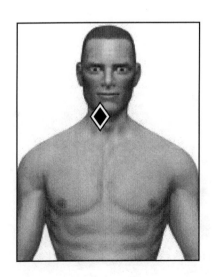
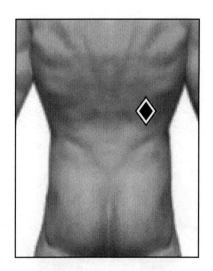

CONTROLS CONVULSIONS
Cerebellum - Cerebellum

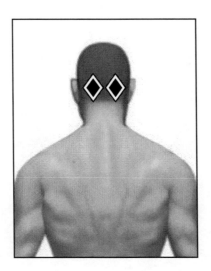

CHRONIC OBSTRUCTIVE PULMONARY DISEASE (COPD)
Thymus - Spleen

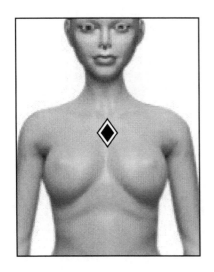
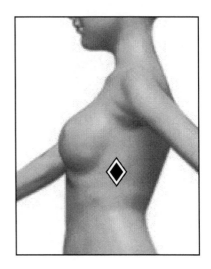

DIGESTIVE/WEIGHT DISORDERS
Iliac - Iliac

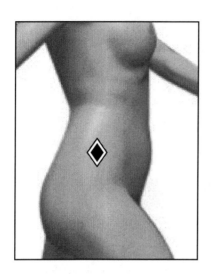 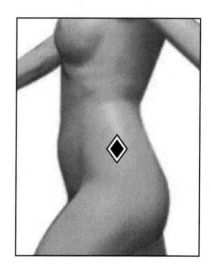

DISTISFACTION FROM ANATOMICAL ALTERATION
(LOSS LIMB, MISCARRIAGE, ABORTION...)
Supraciliary - Oblongata

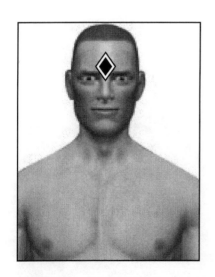 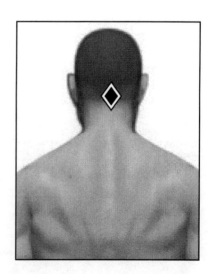

DRUG ADDICTION
Corpus Callosum - Corpus Callosum

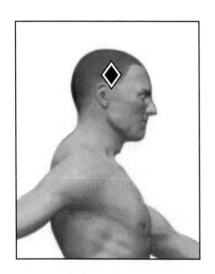 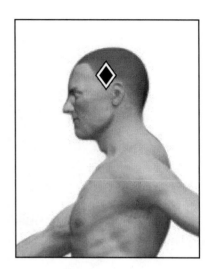

DYSMENORRHEA (PAINFUL MENSTRATION)
Pituitary - Ovary

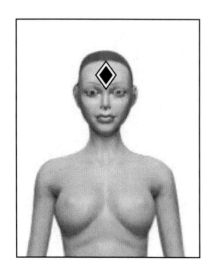 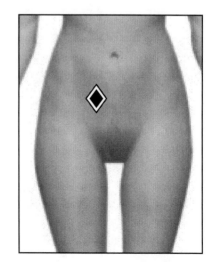

ECTOPIC PREGNANCY
Fallopian - Ovary

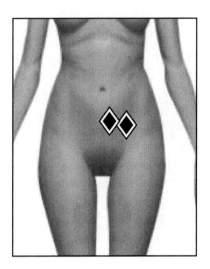

ENERGY BALANCING
Brachial Knot - Brachial Knot

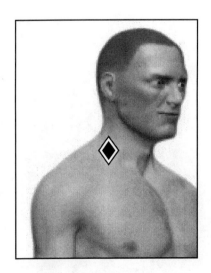 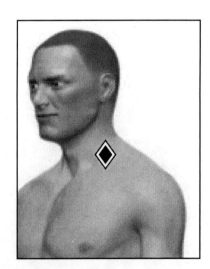

EXCESSIVE APPETITE
Pylorus - Transverse Colon

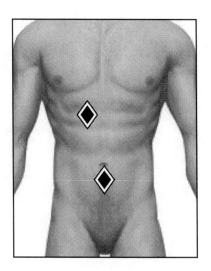

FALSE PREGNANCY
Uterus - Uterus

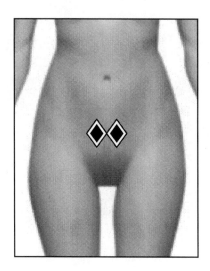

FOOD ALLERGIES
Pancreas - Stomach

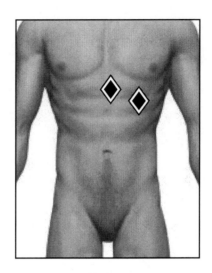

FOOD DETOX
Stomach - Pancreas Tail

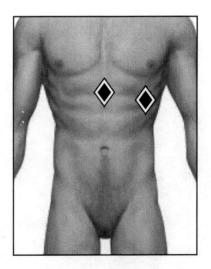

HEAVY METALS INTOXICATION
Pancreas (Head) - Pancreas

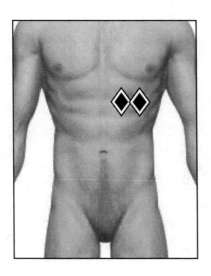

HORMONAL BALANCING
Parotid - Parotid

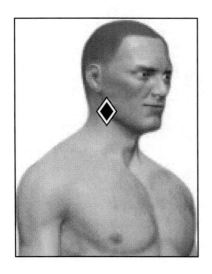 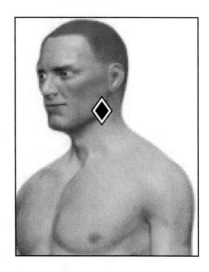

HORMONAL BALANCING
Thymus - Adrenals

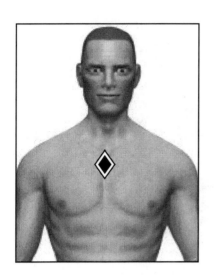 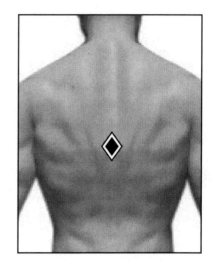

IMMUNODEFICIENCY
Kidney (Superior) - Kidney (Inferior)

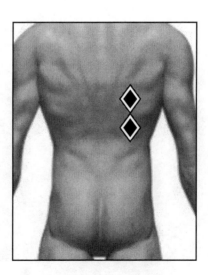

IMPROVES WHITE BLOOD CELL PRODUCTION AND QUALITY. INCREASES LYMPHOCYTES
Thymus - Appendix

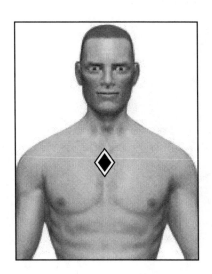 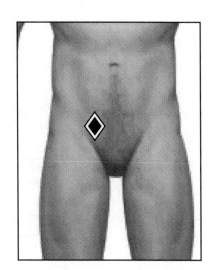

INCREASE PULSE
Oblongata - Heart

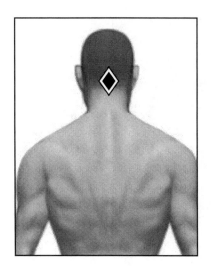 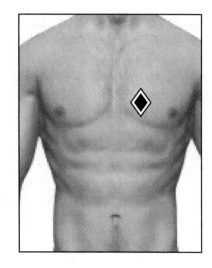

INCREASES LYMPHOCYTES
Appendix - Thymus

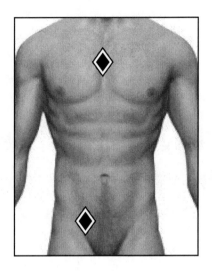

INDICATE PREGNANCY
Uterus - Ovary

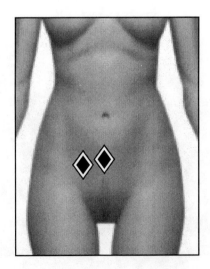

INTESTINAL OBSTRUCTION
Colon (Descending) - Rectum

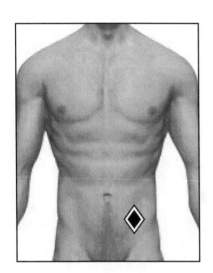
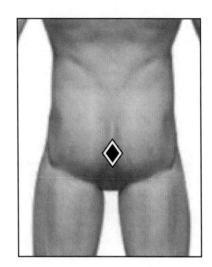

INTOXICATION, NERVOUS TICS
Ear (Cartilage) - Ear (Cartilage)

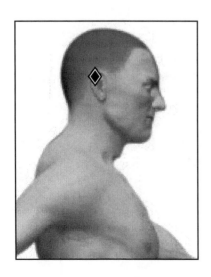
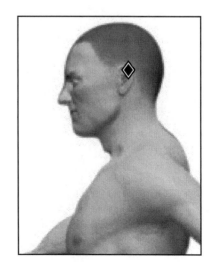

MACULOPATHIES
Macula - Cerebellum

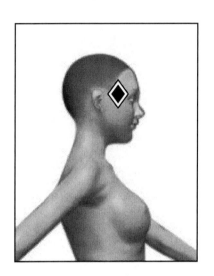
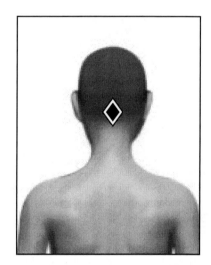

MENSTRUAL CRAMPS, KIDNEY STONES, KIDNEY CRAMPS
Kidney - Ureter

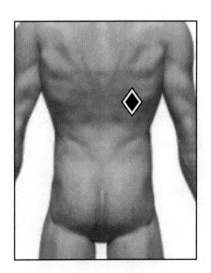
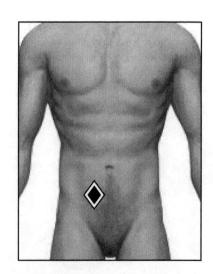

METALLOID INTOXICATION
Liver (Posterior Lobe) - Kidney (Left)

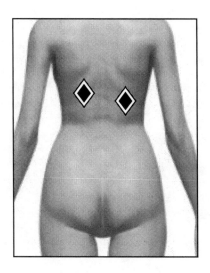

OBESITY
Stomach - Liver

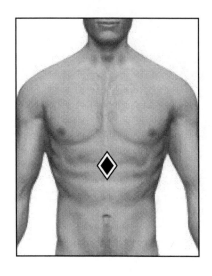
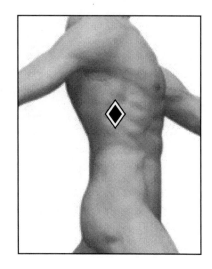

OPTIC NERVE EDEMA
Eye - Cerebellum

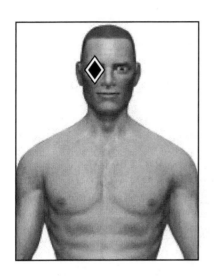 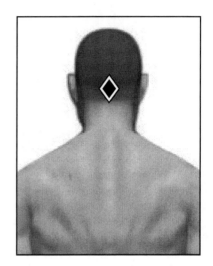

PANCREAS BELT
Pancreas - Pancreas - Pancreas - Pancreas

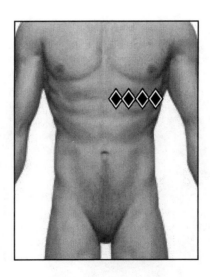

PANCREATITIS
Pancreas - Pancreas

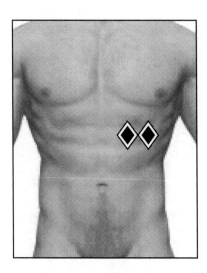

PANCREATITIS
Pancreas Body - Pancreas Tail

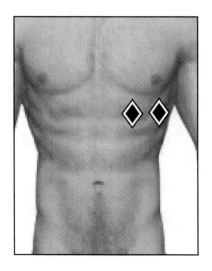

PARASITE RESERVOIR
Stump - Stump

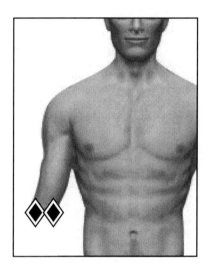

PARKINGSON'S
Post-Pineal - Oblongata

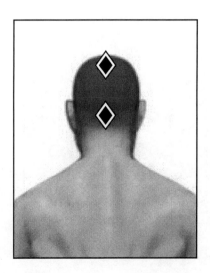

PESTICIDE INTOXICATION
Quadriceps - Quadriceps

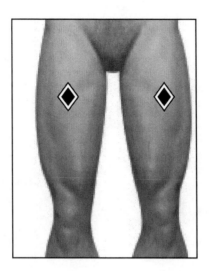

POLYGLOBULIA
Sternum - Adrenals

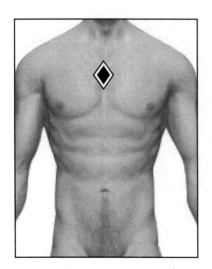 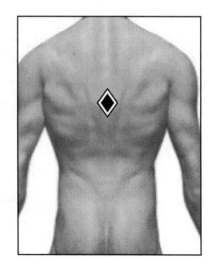

PULMONARY HYPERTENSION
Carotid - Carotid

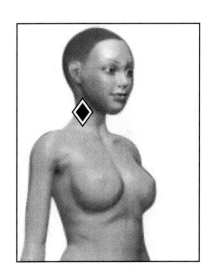 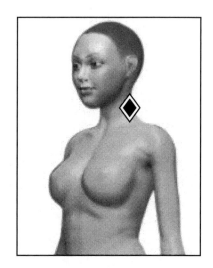

RADICULOPATHY
Paravertebral - Paravertebral

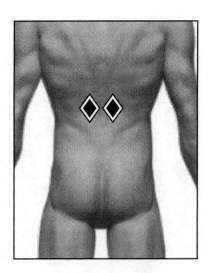

REGULATES LYMPHATIC SYSTEM
Chiasm - Chiasm

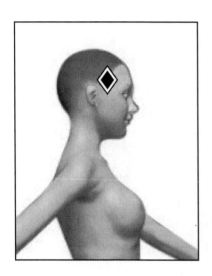 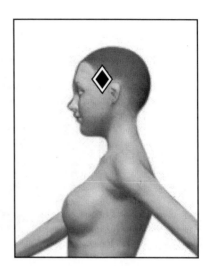

REGULATES SEXUAL LIBIDO (HYPER/HYPO)
Atlas - Atlas

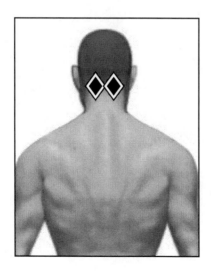

RENAL DYSFUNCTION
Kidney - Renal Capsule (Ipsilateral)

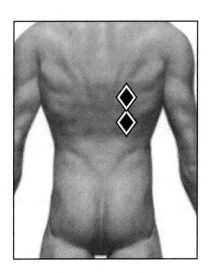

SHORT/LONG LEG
Ear - Kidney (Contralateral)

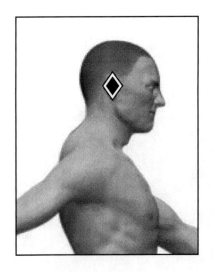
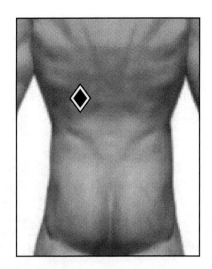

SHORT/LONG LEG
Kidney - Temporal (Contralateral)

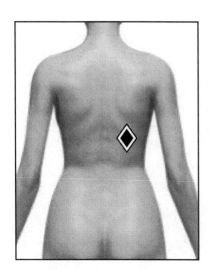
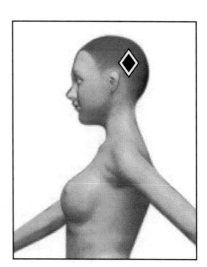

SHORT/LONG LEG
Parietal - Kidney (Contralateral)

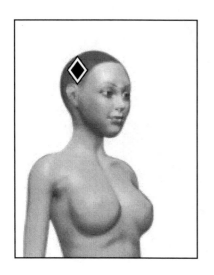
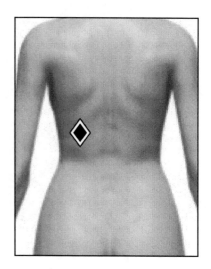

STIMULATES LACTATION
Pineal - Mammary

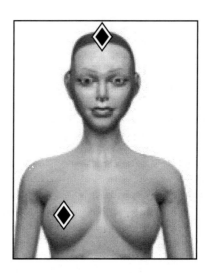

SUFFOCATION
Heart (Inferior Tip) - Ribs (Ipsilateral)

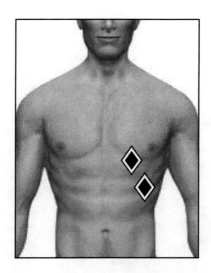

TENIS ELBOW
Cervical (7th) - Thoracic (1st)

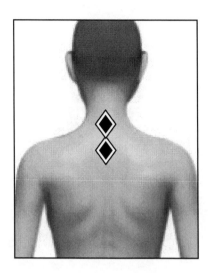

TINNITUS
Mastoides - Kidney (Ipsilateral)

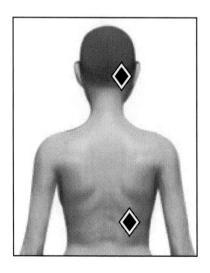

VERTICAL EQUILIBRIUM, DISLEXIA
Frontal Pole - Frontal Pole

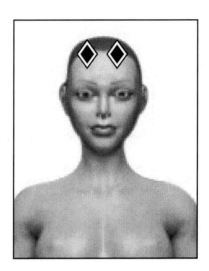

VISUAL DISORDERS, MYOPIA
Elbow - Elbow

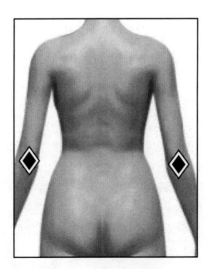

ABOUT RECALIBRATION BIOMAGNETISM

Throughout the years of helping people experience the great benefits of Medical Biomagnetism, Mr. Durazo has been asked several times by people who want to be a part of the biomagnetic mission to teach them this science. For many years, Durazo politely declined because it made better sense for everybody to study directly with the *master* - Dr. Isaac Goiz Durán - himself.

The sad truth is that even though Dr. Goiz did train thousands of people throughout his lifetime, only a small percentage of his students actually practice professionally. It may appear that the three main reasons would-be practitioners quit is because:

1. Although at first glance it many seem easy to learn Medical Biomagnetism, the truth is it requires an incredible amount of time studying and practice.

2. Medical Biomagnetism is virtually unheard of, or misunderstood, so there are issues having to do with educating people. This means that the marketing component is immense, and unless one is really good at communicating, financial struggles cause people to abandon this path, and...

3. Perhaps the most common reason why people give up is because of the responsibility associated with this mission. The healthcare consumer (i.e. the patient) puts enormous responsibility on the practitioner.

For example, Durazo explained to me that in the beginning he would feel a huge weight on his shoulders. Often times, people with serious diagnosis and chronic pain, for example, cancer, would tell him, *"I'm told I have a few months to live, but I know you're going to cure me".*

For the above reasons, coupled with censorship, Medical Pair Biomagnetism remains virtually unheard of. Direct access to a qualified practitioner continues to be challenging.

For many years Durazo wondered how he can best do his part in bringing Biomagnetism directly into people's lives. This is when he started writing books, had an online radio program, delivered weekly biomagnetic Q&A talks at his office, and then finally something happened that helped him see things in a different light. This life changing moment was the beginning of the development of a mind, body, spirit biomagnetic healing approach that he calls *Recalibration Biomagnetism.*

In December of 2015 Durazo saw his toddler son suffer from a severe cough, and within five minutes after giving him a medical biomagnetic treatment he saw the coughing dramatically diminish. His son went from misery, to then energized and playing and smiling like it was bright and early in the day, and nothing was a matter.

This amazing experience made him think of all the miserable pain and suffering in the world in a way he could never understand before becoming a parent. From a mental/intellectual perspective, he had always known that the world would undoubtedly be a better place if more people just knew about and had access to Medical Biomagnetism. But he now understood it in his heart, as a matter of the old cliché: love, peace and harmony. He thought, Biomagnetism MUST be a part of everyone's life - period!

Durazo knew that in order to help more people experience the great benefits of Biomagnetism, we needed a simplified do-it-yourself version that is superior to the limited magnet therapy (i.e. magnetic jewelry, show inserts, mattresses, etc.), and that could yield equal (if not greater) results as Medical Biomagnetism, that anybody, including children, could learn how to use.

Fusing his holistic training with his medical biomagnetic pair knowledge, he developed a six-step protocol, and began testing it with members of his private medical association. This biomagnetic recalibration approach was about applying magnets while specifically focusing on one of six mind, body, spirit challenges and/or solutions per day, with the intention of improving every aspect of one's life.

After much trial and feedback from the initial users, it was interesting to notice how deeply ingrained in our minds is the allopathic approach that there must be a specific-pill per sign and/or symptom, as opposed to looking at the possible underlying life-style habits that lead us to the pain and suffering, and transforming those habits and/or beliefs.

Although users were having great transformational experiences from a mind, body, perspective, the recurring question by those that learned to use Recalibration Biomagnetism is, *"Where do I place the magnets for high blood pressure, diabetes, arthritis, cholesterol, etc.?"* These are valid questions, but if the answer to the above question is all that is important, then that is a limited mind-set.

If we're going to be in great control of our lives, we must also ask, *"How do I diminish my stress levels, improve my nutritional intake, diminish intoxication, improve my relationships, etc...?"* Or, *"What do I need to do to maintain optimal mind, body and spirit fitness?"*

After 20 years in the healthcare system, Durazo has learned that placing great importance on medication, supplements, diets, counseling, therapeutic modalities, religion, politics and other, as the principal solutions to our problems are not the entirety of the solution.

By understanding this general mental limit, it was evident that in order to have a successful do-it-yourself biomagnetic system, it must help us go beyond the notion that pain-relief is the end goal, but rather that optimal mind, body and spirit function is the ultimate goal! In other words, let us not only focus on stopping the problem, but also to live the version of our best life every moment of life!

If your life were perfect, if you could change your circumstances right now, how would your life be different? What would you be doing? How would you feel? What things (perhaps) would you not be doing? It is by asking these questions that we can discover what we truly want in our life and begin to live it. Science shows that happier people are the ones that get sick the least, so doesn't it make the most sense to make joy and other feel-good emotions the objective?

The Recalibration Biomagnetism foundation Durazo developed has to do with identifying both the challenges and solutions of the mind, body and spirit and applying magnets to the body to recalibrate these three bodies.

The recalibrating biomagnetic approach is one that promotes personal alignment to how our lives would be in an ideal world where everything is amazing every moment of life in spite of our daily challenges

– let's call that *perfect*.

This self-awareness component is very powerful. So many people have reported that this written exercise alone helped them see their mental and lifestyle habits that are hindering them, and this helped overcome mind, body and spirit conflicts even without the use of magnets. Of course, when you use magnets, you get greater results for they help stimulate the body to help us function to the best of our abilities.

This recalibrating system delivers:

- Six (6) powerful self-evaluation strategies,
- Six (6) recalibrating biomagnetic formulas,
- Detoxification formula,
- Pain relief formula,
- Immune support formula,
- 11 body systems advanced combinations,
- How to perform distance healing,
- How to bio-energetically muscle test, and more...

By incorporating these powerful tools and techniques, you can optimize your body's natural abilities to heal, restore balance, and enhance overall well-being. The recalibrating system provides targeted formulas for specific health concerns, enabling you to address issues such as pain, immune support, and detoxification.

To complement your journey with the Recalibration Biomagnetism system and further explore the depths of your spiritual health and transformation, I invite you to discover my *Spiritual Thriving* book. This valuable resource offers additional insights, guidance, and specific pendulum-based practices to enhance your spiritual evolution. By combining the power of self-awareness, biomagnetic recalibration, and pendulum work, you can unlock new levels of spiritual thriving and embrace a life of profound well-being.

To learn more about the Biomagnetic Recalibration System books, magnets, and courses, as well as explore the pendulum charts in *Spiritual Thriving*, visit www.SaveMeMagnets.com. Embark on this transformative journey and empower yourself to create lasting positive changes in your health, wisdom, and spiritual growth.

FREQUENTLY ASKED QUESTIONS

1: *Why don't the illustrations in this book show where to place the positive or negative polarities?*

The reason the illustrations are not labeled with positive and negative symbols is because Medical Pair Biomagnetism understands that polarity may differ from person to person. For example, one person may need a negative on the thymus, and a positive on the spleen, while a different person would require the inverse placement. Determining the appropriate polarity requires in-depth training beyond the scope of this book.

However, if you are open-minded and eager to learn and take action, my book, *"Pendulum Charts for Medical Pair Biomagnetism,"* can greatly assist you in mastering the art of diagnosing. This comprehensive guide not only provides efficient guidance in understanding the illustrated pairs needed, but the pendulum charts introduce you to an enhanced use of a pendulum. By asking simple yes/no questions, you can determine the precise polarity required for each placement. With this book as your guide, you can confidently navigate the intricacies of Medical Pair Biomagnetism and achieve optimal results in your practice.

2: *How can I learn to biomagnetically detect a person's pH imbalances, and then correctly apply the magnetic polarities.*

To gain expertise in biomagnetically detecting pH imbalances and accurately applying the magnetic polarities, I recommend visiting *SaveMeMagnets.com.* They offer comprehensive in-person and online courses specifically designed to equip you with the necessary knowledge and skills. Additionally, utilizing the *"Pendulum Charts for Medical Pair Biomagnetism"* book mentioned earlier will further enhance your understanding and practical application of biomagnetic therapy. By combining the valuable resources provided by *SaveMeMagnets.com* and the guidance offered in the book, you will be well on your way to mastering the detection and correction of pH imbalances through the effective use of biomagnetism together with a pendulum.

3: *Are the pairs in this book all of Dr. Goiz' complete pairs, or are there more?*

These pairs were taught by Dr. Goiz because they had completed a research process. When you see publishings of hundreds more pairings, these are conclusions from other practitioners, and they may or may not be verified.

4: *If I had those pairings, would they work?*

The only way to find out is by testing, applying and getting results, and you can learn this process by taking a course at *SaveMeMagnets.com* with specialist Mr. Durazo.

5: *How can I get magnets to get started on Biomagnetism?*

You can get yourself a simple Quick Start Biomagnetic kit, or get the complete Recalibration Biomagnetism system (highly suggested). Go to *SaveMeMagnets.com* for more information.

Suggested Reading & Educational Resources

1. Pendulum Charts For Medical Pair Biomagnetism: Efficient Healing and Targeted Wellness, by Victoria Vivaldi

2. Spiritual Thriving: Navigating Health, Wisdom and Transformation with Pendulum Charts, by Victoria Vivaldi

3. The Power of Self-Care: Using Biomagnetism for Suicide Prevention and Mental Wellness (Co-Authored with Moses Durazo)

4. Biomagnetism: The Mind, Body, Spirit Recalibration System, by Moses Durazo (available as a kit on Amazon)

5. How you can Prevent, Improve and Cure Disease Using Magnets – Goizean Medical Biomagnetism and Bioenergetics: Frequently Asked Questions, by Moses Durazo

6. Medical Magnets: Saving Lives and Millions of Dollars in Healthcare, by Moses Durazo

7. The Courage to Face COVID-19, by John Leake and Peter A. McCullough, MD, MPH

8. The Real Anthony Fauci: Bill Gates, Big Pharma, and the Global War on Democracy and Public Health, by Robert F. Kennedy

9. TheHighwire.com (online investigative journalism)

10. ChildrensHealthDefense.org

Made in the USA
Monee, IL
16 March 2025

14064209R00116